Motivational Interviewing
for
CLINICAL PRACTICE

Motivational Interviewing
for
CLINICAL PRACTICE

Edited by

Petros Levounis, M.D., M.A.
Bachaar Arnaout, M.D.
Carla Marienfeld, M.D.

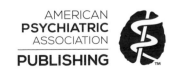

AMERICAN
PSYCHIATRIC
ASSOCIATION
PUBLISHING

If you wish to buy 50 or more copies of the same title, please go to www.appi.org/specialdiscounts for more information.

Copyright © 2017 American Psychiatric Association Publishing

ALL RIGHTS RESERVED
First Edition
Manufactured in the United States of America on acid-free paper
21   5   4   3   2

American Psychiatric Association Publishing
1000 Wilson Boulevard
Arlington, VA 22209-3901
www.appi.org

Library of Congress Cataloging-in-Publication Data
Names: Levounis, Petros, editor. | Arnaout, Bachaar, 1974- editor. | Marienfeld, Carla, editor.
Title: Motivational interviewing for clinical practice / edited by Petros Levounis, Bachaar Arnaout, Carla Marienfeld.
Description: First edition. | Arlington, Virginia : American Psychiatric Association Publishing, [2017] | Includes bibliographical references and index.
Identifiers: LCCN 2016051307 (print) | LCCN 2016052639 (ebook) | ISBN 9781615370467 (pbk. : alk. paper) | ISBN 9781615371242 ()
Subjects: | MESH: Motivational Interviewing | Interview, Psychological
Classification: LCC RC454 (print) | LCC RC454 (ebook) | NLM WM 55 | DDC 616.89—dc23
LC record available at https://lccn.loc.gov/2016051307

British Library Cataloguing in Publication Data
A CIP record is available from the British Library.

Contents

Part 1
Getting Ready to
Use Motivational Interviewing

Part 2
Getting Good at
Motivational Interviewing

Part 3
Getting Advanced Knowledge in
Motivational Interviewing

Contributors

Michelle C. Acosta, Ph.D.
Principal Investigator and Administrative Director, Center for Technology and Health, National Development and Research Institutes, Inc., New York, New York

Elie G. Aoun, M.D.
Addiction Psychiatry Fellow, Department of Psychiatry, University of California, San Francisco, San Francisco, California

Bachaar Arnaout, M.D.
Assistant Professor of Psychiatry, Yale School of Medicine, VA Connecticut Healthcare System, West Haven, Connecticut

Angela R. Bethea-Walsh, Ph.D.
Licensed Psychologist, Bethea Consulting and Psychological Services, P.C., Atlanta, Georgia

Curtis Bone, M.D., M.H.S.
Addiction Medicine Fellow, Yale School of Medicine, New Haven, Connecticut

Noah Capurso, M.D., M.H.S.
Assistant Professor of Psychiatry, Yale School of Medicine, New Haven, Connecticut

Jeffrey DeVido, M.D., M.T.S.
Assistant Professor, Department of Psychiatry, University of California, San Francisco School of Medicine, San Francisco, California

Deborah L. Haller, Ph.D.
Voluntary Associate Professor, Department of Public Health Sciences, Miller School of Medicine, University of Miami, Miami, Florida

Brian Hurley, M.D., M.B.A., DFASAM
Robert Wood Johnson Foundation Clinical Scholar, David Geffen School of Medicine, University of California, Los Angeles, Los Angeles, California

Ayana Jordan, M.D., Ph.D.
Assistant Professor, Department of Psychiatry, Yale School of Medicine, New Haven, Connecticut

Vicki Kalira, M.D.
Assistant Clinical Professor, New York University Langone Medical Center, New York

SueAnn Kim, M.D.
Addiction Psychiatry Fellow, New York University School of Medicine, New York

Grace Kwon, D.O.
Addiction Psychiatry Fellow, Department of Psychiatry, Yale School of Medicine, New Haven, Connecticut

Petros Levounis, M.D., M.A.
Professor and Chair, Department of Psychiatry, Rutgers New Jersey Medical School; Chief of Service, University Hospital, Newark, New Jersey

Marie-Josée Lynch, M.D., C.M.
Addiction Psychiatry Fellow, Department of Psychiatry, Yale School of Medicine, New Haven, Connecticut

Carla Marienfeld, M.D.
Associate Professor of Psychiatry, University of California, San Diego, San Diego, California

Steve Martino, Ph.D.
Professor of Psychiatry, Yale School of Medicine, New Haven; Chief, Psychology Service, VA Connecticut Healthcare System, West Haven, Connecticut

Teofilo E. Matos Santana, M.D.
Assistant Professor, Department of Psychiatry, Yale School of Medicine, New Haven, Connecticut

Edward V. Nunes, M.D.
Professor of Psychiatry, Columbia University and New York State Psychiatric Institute; Principal Investigator, Greater New York Node, National Drug Abuse Clinical Trials Network, New York State Psychiatric Institute, New York

Caridad C. Ponce Martinez, M.D.
Assistant Professor of Psychiatry, University of Massachusetts Medical School, Worcester, Massachusetts; Assistant Professor Adjunct of Psychiatry, Yale School of Medicine, New Haven, Connecticut

Richard N. Rosenthal, M.D.
Professor of Psychiatry, Icahn School of Medicine at Mount Sinai, New York

Mandrill Taylor, M.D., M.P.H.
Addiction Psychiatry Fellow, Department of Psychiatry, Yale School of Medicine, New Haven, Connecticut

Students and Residents

David L. Convissar, M.D.
Rutgers New Jersey Medical School 2016; Rutgers Anesthesiology 2020

Isaac Johnson
Yale School of Medicine, MS2

Jill Konowich, Ph.D.
Rutgers New Jersey Medical School, MS-IV

David Kopel
Rutgers New Jersey Medical School, MS-IV

Jose Medina, M.S.W.
Rutgers New Jersey Medical School, MS-II

Eli Neustadter
Yale School of Medicine, MS2

Emmanuel Ohuabunwa, M.D., M.B.A. candidate
Yale School of Medicine, MS4

Anil Rengan
Rutgers New Jersey Medical School, MS-IV

Amy Schettino
Yale School of Medicine, MS3

Augustine Tawadros
Rutgers New Jersey Medical School, MS-III

Melissa Thomas
Yale School of Medicine, MS2

Mike Wang
Yale School of Medicine, MS3

Disclosure of Competing Interests

The following contributors to this book have indicated a financial interest in or other affiliation with a commercial supporter, a manufacturer of a commercial product, a provider of a commercial service, a nongovernmental organization, and/or a government agency, as listed below:

Jeffrey DeVido, M.D., M.T.S.—*Shareholder:* Altria; Phillip Morris Co. (neither of which are specific focus of the author's contributions).

The following contributors to this book have no competing interests to report:

Michelle C. Acosta, Ph.D.
Elie G. Aoun, M.D.
Bachaar Arnaout, M.D.
Angela R. Bethea-Walsh, Ph.D.
Curtis Bone, M.D., M.H.S.
Deborah L. Haller, Ph.D.
Brian Hurley, M.D., M.B.A., DFASAM
Ayana Jordan, M.D., Ph.D.
Vicki Kalira, M.D.
SueAnn Kim, M.D.
Grace Kwon, D.O.
Marie-Josée Lynch, M.D., C.M.
Petros Levounis, M.D., M.A.
Carla Marienfeld, M.D.
Steve Martino, Ph.D.
Teofilo E. Matos Santana, M.D.
Caridad C. Ponce Martinez, M.D.

Preface

This is a book about celebrating and resolving ambivalence.

When American Psychiatric Association Publishing asked us to update our 2010 *Handbook of Motivation and Change: A Practical Guide for Clinicians,* we were, well, ambivalent. On one hand, we were quite pleased with our 2010 little labor of love. On the other hand, things have changed in the world of motivational interviewing (MI) over the past half dozen years.

We now welcome the opportunity to spruce up our 2010 ideas and introduce new concepts and techniques and new ways of presenting MI throughout our new book. We've changed the title and—more importantly—added a third editor. We are thrilled that Carla Marienfeld has joined our MI adventures.

This book is a practical resource for the busy clinician. For this new book, we aimed for a book that is informative, very practical, easy to read, and fun! Our audience is primarily the general psychiatrist or clinician with no particular expertise (and sometimes not even particular interest) in addiction treatment. However, we hope that this book will also be helpful to family practitioners, internists, pediatricians, medical students, allied professionals, and anyone else who may be interested in issues of motivation and change.

The main theoretical platform for our book is *motivational interviewing,* as described by William R. Miller and Stephen Rollnick (2013) in their book *Motivational Interviewing: Helping People Change,* 3rd Edition. However, we open the theoretical framework to include other ideas and techniques that therapists and counselors may have found helpful in their scholarship and everyday clinical experience.

The book is organized in three parts:

Part 1: Getting Ready to Use Motivational Interviewing
Part 2: Getting Good at Motivational Interviewing
Part 3: Getting Advanced Knowledge in Motivational Interviewing

In the current book, we have replaced most of the case studies in the 2010 book with examples of clinical dialogue, which we have found to be most useful to both novices and experts. We have also included as many clinical tools—such as flow sheets and summary tables—as possible to bring the material to life. Key points, references, and multiple-choice examination questions with explanation of the correct answers complete the educational mission of this book.

At the end of the each chapter, we have added a new feature: feedback from learners new to MI. We asked six medical students from Rutgers New Jersey Medical School and six medical students from Yale School of Medicine (our academic homes) to read a chapter and describe in a few paragraphs what they think will be most useful to them in the future. Their responses have educated, surprised, and thoroughly delighted us.

From the medical students to the trainees, our colleagues, our patients, and our mentors, we are profoundly grateful for the support—and inspiration—that we have received. We are also greatly indebted to our loved ones: Petros would like to thank his husband, Lukas; Bachaar, his parents, Barbara and Saad, and his children, Nadia and Sophia; and Carla, her husband, Juan, and daughter, Julia. Thank you for motivating us every day to keep resolving ambivalence and celebrating life.

Petros Levounis, M.D., M.A.

Bachaar Arnaout, M.D.

Carla Marienfeld, M.D.

Newark, New Jersey, and New Haven, Connecticut
Summer 2016

Getting Ready to Use Motivational Interviewing

Motivational Interviewing in Addiction Treatment

Edward V. Nunes, M.D.

How do we talk with patients? As physicians and psychiatrists, having made a diagnostic assessment and a treatment plan, how do we get our patients to follow it? Surprisingly little in medical school or specialty training, even psychiatric training, teaches us to do this well, even though it would seem a rather fundamental clinical skill. The same may often be true in allied fields such as psychology, social work, and nursing. There is a focus during training in medical school on patient-centered interviewing. But *motivational interviewing* (MI) is more than a patient-centered interview. It is a patient-centered effort to help patients change their health behaviors, and that is more challenging. To help patients change behavior, we should pay more attention to MI, read this book and others, respect the task, and practice and develop our skills.

Medical and psychiatric training focus on biology, psychology, disease mechanisms, and treatment methods. The assumption is that patients, having received an explanation and a recommendation, will naturally fall into line and follow the recommended course of therapy. Yet, failure to adhere to recommended treatments is common across a wide range of illnesses, from medical problems such as hypertension or management of cardiovascular risk factors (e.g., diet, exercise) to psychiatric disorders, including substance use disorders. In a broader sense, the methods and skills of MI can be applied to any health behavior that one is trying to get a patient to follow, be it giving up alcohol, giving up cigarettes, taking medication for hypertension or high cholesterol, or changing dietary and exercise habits. A large proportion of national disease burden in developed countries can be traced to such health behaviors. Yet, as clinicians well know, these behaviors are hard to change, and it is often not enough to simply tell patients it is time to quit alcohol or cigarettes or make other changes in lifestyle, or to adhere to treatments that may be cumbersome or uncomfortable in one way or another.

The development of new treatments for substance dependence has been an intensive focus of research over the past four decades, accelerated by a growing awareness of the morbidity and social costs of the addictions, including addiction to nicotine, alcohol, and other drugs. This investment in research has produced a number of promising medications and psychotherapeutic and behavioral treatments with solid evidence of efficacy from clinical trials. Medications include methadone, buprenorphine, and naltrexone (including injectable naltrexone) for opioid dependence; disulfiram, naltrexone, and acamprosate for alcohol dependence; and nicotine replacement, bupropion, and varenicline for nicotine dependence. Behavioral approaches include various cognitive-behavioral and family therapy approaches, 12-step facilitation, and contingency management using vouchers or prizes as rewards for abstinence. Further, important treatment approaches have been developed out of experience and clinical work, including 12-step methods such as Alcoholics Anonymous and various residential treatment approaches such as the 28-day model and long-term therapeutic community treatment. Evidence supporting the effectiveness of many of these treatments abounds. For example, the National Institute on Drug Abuse (NIDA) Clinical Trials Network has been engaged in testing evidence-based treatments when delivered by clinicians in real-world, community-based treatment settings, and has found considerable support for the effectiveness of such treatments, both behavioral (e.g., Ball et al. 2007; Carroll et al. 2006; Donovan et al. 2013; Hien et al. 2010; Peirce et al. 2006; Petry et al. 2005; Tross et al. 2008) and pharmacological (Hser et al. 2014; Weiss et al. 2011). All told, the scope of progress has been considerable.

Among all these treatment approaches, MI is of special importance because it can be viewed as the essential clinical skill for engaging patients in treatment and motivating patients to reduce substance use and to follow through with specific behavioral or pharmacological treatments recommended. It is also challenging to master. It requires restraining old tendencies such as asking lots of closed-ended questions, telling patients what to do, or confronting patients who don't follow recommendations. Such tendencies are fairly typical in medical encounters with patients in the effort to rapidly arrive at a diagnosis and treatment plan. MI also involves learning sophisticated new skills, such as using reflections instead of closed-ended questions, using complex reflections, and using the tactical combination of open-ended questions, reflections, and summarizations to move the patient toward change.

EFFICACY OF MOTIVATIONAL INTERVIEWING

Controlled Trials and Meta-analyses

MI enjoys extensive evidence of efficacy from controlled trials in alcohol (e.g., Bien et al. 1993; Borsari and Carey 2000; Marlatt et al. 1998; Miller et al. 1993; Project MATCH Research Group 1997) and drug use disorders (Babor et al. 1999; Ball et al. 2007; Carroll et al. 2006; Martino et al. 2000; Saunders et al. 1995; Swanson et al. 1999). Several meta-analyses of clinical trials of MI for alcohol, drugs, and other problem health behaviors confirm overall modest effect sizes. The meta-analyses also highlight variability of effect across populations, settings, and types of clinicians, as well as variability in the methodological quality of the trials (Burke et al. 2003; Hettema et al. 2005; Li et al. 2016; Smedslund et al. 2011).

Importance of Skill in Motivational Interviewing

Efforts to delineate the underlying mechanisms of MI have examined the relationship between particular therapist behaviors or skills on engendering change in patients, and these have direct implications for how to design training methods for MI. A seminal finding has been that when a patient makes statements during an MI session committing to changing his or her behavior (a.k.a. *commitment language,* or *change talk*), this is associated with improved substance use outcomes at follow-up (Amrhein et al. 2003; Moyers et al. 2007). Further, evidence suggests that therapist behavior consistent with MI is more likely to engender change talk, while MI-inconsistent behavior (e.g., directing, confronting) is associated with expressions of resistance to change (*counter change talk,* or *sustain talk*) (Moyers and Martin 2006; Moyers et al. 2007). Other studies have examined the relative importance of clinicians' specific MI-consistent behaviors and skills (e.g., affirming, asking open-ended questions, making reflections) versus a more global interpersonal style or the spirit of MI (e.g., collaborativeness, empathy). Findings have tended to show that the global skills and spirit of MI may be more powerful than the specific skills in engendering client engagement and treatment alliance (Boardman et al. 2006; Moyers et al. 2005), although these latter studies did not assess change talk among patients. The implications for training include the following: 1) it is important to teach clinicians MI-consistent behaviors and to minimize MI-inconsistent behaviors, with an emphasis on teaching the global style and spirit of MI; and 2) clinicians should be trained to recognize and reinforce their patients' change talk.

BASIC PRINCIPLES OF
MOTIVATIONAL INTERVIEWING

In medical school and residency training, physicians learn to conduct diagnostic evaluations, order tests, and prescribe medications and other treatments. In a sense, the emphasis is on a model of the physician, bedecked with a white coat, as the authority. And, after so many years of training, you develop expertise. The same may apply to training in psychology and other allied health fields. Even in clinical training, such as psychiatric residency, where psychotherapy is taught, many of the specific psychotherapeutic techniques can take on the same authoritative stance. In cognitive-behavioral approaches, for example, the therapist is in the role of a teacher, providing formulations regarding patterns of thought and behavior that need to be changed and giving out homework assignments.

Motivational interviewing (Miller and Rollnick 2002, 2013) is founded partly on the clinical intuition of its founders and partly on psychological research, which shows that when a person is ambivalent about making a particular change in his or her behavior, a prescriptive approach is likely to engender resistance and to decrease the probability of change. Hence, giving orders and prescribing changes in behavior, as we have been taught to do, may often be countertherapeutic. Instead, people are more likely to change when it is their own free decision, for reasons that they have determined and endorsed.

MI is also founded on the theory of *cognitive dissonance*. When a person holds conflicting ideas in their mind, it creates dissonance, and there is a tendency to resolve the conflict in one direction or the other. For a patient with drug or alcohol dependence, there are usually many unpleasant facts about the consequences of the substance use, which, if viewed starkly, are at odds with the person's deeply held values and what he or she cares about. The effort in MI is to help the patient to view such facts starkly, while at the same time elicit the patient's deeply held values, in order to elicit and amplify the cognitive dissonance between the two and create a drive for change. This resolution of cognitive dissonance could go either way in the sense that the person could decide to change his or her behavior and stop using substances, or conversely, to reframe or minimize the facts and continue using substances. The skill of the therapist is to guide the patient toward internally motivated change.

In the second edition of their central text on MI, Miller and Rollnick (2002) defined what they called the "spirit" of MI, describing a way of being with and talking with patients founded on collaboration, evocation, and autonomy.

- *Collaboration:* The patient should be approached as a partner in a consultative manner. The emphasis is on working together with the patient to arrive at decisions as to what to do and how to proceed. This is the opposite of the classic authoritative, prescriptive stance that we clinicians tend to inherit from our basic training.

- *Evocation:* The clinician should ask the patient about what is important to him or her, what he or she values, and then listen carefully and formulate further questions mainly to further draw out the patient's point of view. Thus, the emphasis is on open-ended questions and active, "reflective" listening. This is the opposite of the intensive fact-finding and closed-ended questions that are characteristic of the typical diagnostic interview.
- *Autonomy:* The patient is ultimately in charge of his or her care, and the clinician should respect the patient's decisions and freedom to choose. This is the opposite of the paternalistic stance of clinician as teacher and authority figure.

In the third edition of their central text, Miller and Rollnick (2013) refined and expanded the dimensions of the spirit of MI to include partnership, acceptance, compassion, and evocation.

- *Partnership:* Similar to the notion of collaboration, the patient should be approached as a partner in a consultative manner. The emphasis is on working together with the patient to arrive at decisions as to what to do and how to proceed, rather than assuming the classic authoritative, prescriptive stance often characteristic of clinicians. The authors liken MI to "dancing rather than wrestling" with the patient. This also involves recognizing that the clinician will have an agenda for the patient (to stop using drugs or alcohol typically), but the patient's agenda must be respected as well, and it is ultimately the patient who must decide to implement change.
- *Acceptance:* Acceptance, founded in the work of Carl Rogers, is further divided into four concepts: *absolute worth*, involving valuing and accepting the patient for who they are, as opposed to passing judgment; *accurate empathy*, the effort to deeply understand the patient's point of view without allowing the clinician's perspective to interfere; *autonomy support*, respecting that the patient is in charge and needs to decide for himself or herself the course of action, as opposed to any attempt by the clinician to impose on or coerce the patient toward particular goals; and *affirmation*, identifying and recognizing a patient's strengths, abilities, and efforts, rather than focusing on weaknesses or failures.
- *Compassion:* Compassion here means a fundamental commitment to understand and pursue the best interests of the patient. This is emphasized to ensure that MI is intended to support the goals and values of the patient, not those of the clinician or anyone else.
- *Evocation:* Evocation reflects a fundamental assumption of MI: that the patient has strengths and capabilities and that the goal is to draw these out. This is in contrast to a deficit model that pervades much of medicine and other

clinical work—namely, that the patient lacks something or has weaknesses, which the therapy will seek to build or strengthen.

These are not entirely new ideas. For example, informed consent, which has emerged in recent decades as a cornerstone of medical care, holds that patients should be fully informed by their physicians and be a partner in making decisions about how to proceed with their care. This tenet grows out of the medical ethical principle of "respect for persons" and respect for the autonomy of the individual. It is an ethical imperative, but there is also the recognition that patients are more likely to cooperate, and the clinical outcome is likely to be better, if patients are, in fact, active partners in their own care, rather than passive recipients, as in the "doctor knows best" model. Indeed, this has probably been one of the basic components of good "bedside manner" long before the articulations of medical ethics or MI.

What Motivational Interviewing Is Not

These principles would be familiar to any good salesman. However, it is emphasized that MI is not intended to persuade a patient to move in a direction that is not of their choosing, to get the patient to do what the clinician wants, or to coerce the patient. A good salesman uses techniques that are similar to MI. A good salesman gets to know the customer to understand the customer's interests and priorities. The salesman can then describe his or her company's products in light of how they would fit into the customer's life. The salesman guides the customer toward a decision to buy something. Ideally this helps the customer to purchase a product that will best suit the customer's needs and with which he or she will be most satisfied. We are not taught salesmanship in clinical training, and yet as clinicians we are often placed in the position of promoting treatments and lifestyle changes that patients are not sure that they want. But again, it is important to note that MI is part of medicine that respects autonomy, and for change to occur, it is more likely if it is something the patient wants (Miller and Rollnick 2009). Rather, the effort is to engender internally motivated change—to help the patient articulate what he or she genuinely wants and values, and how the treatment recommendation will help to achieve those aims.

It is also important to recognize that MI is not just a sympathetic ear, or a "client-centered" approach where one listens to the patient and helps the patient decide what to do. It is an active persuasion technique. The clinician has a definite agenda, namely, changing health behavior in the direction of health. The clinician needs to help the patient clarify what he or she values, and how substance use or other health behaviors are getting in the way of those values and ability to change. There is something of a paradox here. As clinicians we promote health and fight disease. But, MI teaches us that to best promote health, we need to help patients discover the health that *they* seek and value.

It is important to recognize that there are situations where the approach of MI is not appropriate (see Miller and Rollnick 2002, Chapter 12, on ethical considerations). Sometimes the situation is urgent, and family members, friends, and clinicians need to bring the patient for acute treatment. A patient who is grossly intoxicated needs to be protected until his or her sobriety and judgment return. A patient who is acutely suicidal needs to be hospitalized, against his or her will if necessary. Where to draw such a line with addicted patients can be less clear. When is the drinking or drug use of a minor teenager so out of control that the parents should exercise their legal authority and force the youngster into residential treatment? When should an adult patient be the subject of an intervention by friends and family? These are difficult judgments, of which a clinician needs always to be mindful.

Motivational Interviewing and the Tradition of Confrontation in Addiction Treatment

Denial and confrontation of denial are two concepts that had been fundamental to the clinical approach to the treatment of addictions. Patients often do seem to deny or minimize the problems caused by an addiction. The traditional idea was that denial needed to be recognized and confronted. The patient needed to be shown the problems and told what to do. If the patient did not take the advice, then perhaps the patient was "not ready," and the clinician might ask the patient to return "when ready." However, it is likely that, once a patient presents at the office of a psychiatrist or other clinician for consultation, more than a few friends and relatives, and perhaps other clinicians, will have already spoken in this way to the patient, perhaps repeatedly. Such an approach is likely to only increase the resistance to change. MI encourages the clinician in this situation, as a first step, to listen to the patient and hear the patient's point of view. Rather than deep denial, what is more likely to emerge is ambivalence. The patient is aware of the problems caused by the addiction and wants to quit, but at the same time there are aspects of the substance, and the taking of the substance, that also attract the patient. MI provides a way to help the patient resolve this ambivalence in the direction of abstinence and health.

MASTERING MOTIVATIONAL INTERVIEWING

MI is not easy to learn. Physicians and other clinicians emerge from professional training, as noted previously, with a lot of knowledge and a tendency to want to impart that knowledge—to teach, recommend, and prescribe, and perhaps even confront. In contrast, the skills of MI require that the clinician forbear and hold these tendencies at bay. This can be surprisingly difficult.

In fact, new skills of all sorts can be surprisingly difficult to impart to clinicians. A substantial literature on continuing medical education (CME) has shown that the usual methods of imparting new knowledge—grand rounds and other lectures, scientific papers, books, and even conferences and workshops—are generally ineffective at actually getting physicians to adopt new treatment techniques. Physicians tend to go back to their offices and clinics and do the same old things. More successful are training programs that incorporate not only such didactic training but also practice with supervision and feedback (Davis 1998; Davis et al. 1992, 1995; Grol 2001). There are two potential barriers: the new treatment is unfamiliar, and it may be difficult. MI is both unfamiliar (to traditionally trained physicians, for example) and difficult (in the sense that some of the concepts may be easy, but the mastery requires time and continued practice).

Research comparing the effectiveness of training methods for substance abuse treatments has begun to emerge. One review (Walters et al. 2005) located 17 such studies that evaluated training mainly for either MI or cognitive-behavioral therapies. The conclusions were that workshops may result in transient improvements in skill but that, mirroring the findings from CME, trainings that involved follow-up after the workshop, including various forms of practice with supervision or feedback, appear to be more effective in engendering lasting skills (Miller et al. 2004; Morgenstern et al. 2001a, 2001b; Sholomskas et al. 2005). More recent work affirms this point—that supervision, or some form of coaching and feedback, is needed to sustain and further augment gains in skill at MI after an initial workshop training (Schwalbe et al. 2014; Smith et al. 2012).

This has important implications for the readers of this book, namely, that reading a book like this is only a start. It is important to learn about MI from didactic sources. This will increase knowledge. This book is intended to serve as such an introduction. The authoritative texts by Miller and Rollnick (2002, 2013) are also recommended. These provide broad introductions to the theory and practice of MI and form the basis for most formal workshops and training programs. The present text is oriented especially toward physicians and other clinicians.

However, to truly learn MI, it is important to get feedback and supervision. Workshops in MI will generally involve role-playing exercises with feedback from the instructor. This is a start, but even participating in these exercises is not the same as seeing patients and receiving feedback and supervision on one's actual clinical interviewing. Thus, readers are encouraged to study this book, then to seek out training that involves making audiotapes of one's interviews and having the opportunity to discuss the interviews with an expert supervisor. The MI Network of Trainers (MINT; www.motivationalinterviewing.org/trainer-listing) is one place to start in locating such experts with whom to work. The Clinical Trials Network, in collaboration with the Addiction Technology Transfer Centers, has also developed training resources for MI (i.e., Motivational Interviewing Assessment: Supervisory Tools for Enhancing Proficiency [MIA:STEP]; www.attcnetwork.org/explore/priorityareas/science/blendinginitiative/miastep/product_materials.asp).

The social costs of the addictions are massive in terms of the suffering of patients and their loved ones and the costs in adverse health effects and associated medical treatments, lost productivity, accidents, and death. The addictions represent only one example out of a larger set of adverse health behaviors (poor diet, sedentary lifestyle, and difficulties with weight control being other examples). Our society now confronts spiraling costs of health care and needs to find a way to control them. Greater emphasis is needed on preventive health care and on helping patients to give up destructive substance use and to make other changes toward healthier lifestyles. Thus, physicians and other clinicians need to be more adept at helping our patients to decide to make these changes and adhere to them. We need to be more effective at motivating our patients toward healthy behavior. MI is, arguably, the essential skill for helping patients to change, and it should be part of the armamentarium of every clinician.

REFERENCES

Amrhein PC, Miller WR, Yahne CE, et al: Client commitment language during motivational interviewing predicts drug use outcomes. J Consult Clin Psychol 71(5):862–878, 2003 14516235

Babor T, McRee B, Stephens RS, et al: Marijuana Treatment Project: overview and results (abstract). Symposium conducted at the Annual Meeting of the American Public Health Association. Chicago, IL, November 1999

Ball SA, Martino S, Nich C, et al: Site matters: multisite randomized trial of motivational enhancement therapy in community drug abuse clinics. J Consult Clin Psychol 75(4):556–567, 2007 17663610

Bien TH, Miller WR, Boroughs JM: Motivational interviewing with alcohol outpatients. Behavioural and Cognitive Psychotherapy 21(4):347–356, 1993

Boardman T, Catley D, Grobe JE, et al: Using motivational interviewing with smokers: do therapist behaviors relate to engagement and therapeutic alliance? J Subst Abuse Treat 31(4):329–339, 2006 17084786

Borsari B, Carey KB: Effects of a brief motivational intervention with college student drinkers. J Consult Clin Psychol 68(4):728–733, 2000 10965648

Burke BL, Arkowitz H, Menchola M: The efficacy of motivational interviewing: a meta-analysis of controlled clinical trials. J Consult Clin Psychol 71(5):843–861, 2003 14516234

Carroll KM, Ball SA, Nich C, et al: Motivational interviewing to improve treatment engagement and outcome in individuals seeking treatment for substance abuse: a multisite effectiveness study. Drug Alcohol Depend 81(3):301–312, 2006 16169159

Davis D: Does CME work? An analysis of the effect of educational activities on physician performance or health care outcomes. Int J Psychiatry Med 28(1):21–39, 1998 9617647

Davis DA, Thomson MA, Oxman AD, et al: Evidence for the effectiveness of CME. A review of 50 randomized controlled trials. JAMA 268(9):1111–1117, 1992 1501333

Davis DA, Thomson MA, Oxman AD, et al: Changing physician performance. A systematic review of the effect of continuing medical education strategies. JAMA 274(9):700–705, 1995 7650822

Donovan DM, Daley DC, Brigham GS, et al: Stimulant abuser groups to engage in 12-step: a multisite trial in the National Institute on Drug Abuse Clinical Trials Network. J Subst Abuse Treat 44(1):103–114, 2013 22657748

Grol R: Improving the quality of medical care: building bridges among professional pride, payer profit, and patient satisfaction. JAMA 286(20):2578–2585, 2001 11722272

Hettema J, Steele J, Miller WR: Motivational interviewing. Annu Rev Clin Psychol 1:91–111, 2005 17716083

Hien DA, Jiang H, Campbell AN, et al: Do treatment improvements in PTSD severity affect substance use outcomes? A secondary analysis from a randomized clinical trial in NIDA's Clinical Trials Network. Am J Psychiatry 167(1):95–101, 2010 19917596

Hser YI, Saxon AJ, Huang D, et al: Treatment retention among patients randomized to buprenorphine/naloxone compared to methadone in a multi-site trial. Addiction 109(1):79–87, 2014 23961726

Li L, Zhu S, Tse N, et al: Effectiveness of motivational interviewing to reduce illicit drug use in adolescents: a systematic review and meta-analysis. Addiction 111(5):795–805, 2016 26687544

Marlatt GA, Baer JS, Kivlahan DR, et al: Screening and brief intervention for high-risk college student drinkers: results from a 2-year follow-up assessment. J Consult Clin Psychol 66(4):604–615, 1998

Martino S, Carroll KM, O'Malley SS, et al: Motivational interviewing with psychiatrically ill substance abusing patients. Am J Addict 9(1):88–91, 2000 10914297

Miller WR, Rollnick S: Motivational Interviewing: Preparing People for Change, 2nd Edition. New York, Guilford, 2002

Miller WR, Rollnick S: Ten things that motivational interviewing is not. Behav Cogn Psychother 37(2):129–140, 2009 19364414

Miller WR, Rollnick S: Motivational Interviewing: Helping People Change, 3rd Edition. New York, Guilford, 2013

Miller WR, Benefield RG, Tonigan JS: Enhancing motivation for change in problem drinking: a controlled comparison of two therapist styles. J Consult Clin Psychol 61(3):455–461, 1993 8326047

Miller WR, Yahne CE, Moyers TB, et al: A randomized trial of methods to help clinicians learn motivational interviewing. J Consult Clin Psychol 72(6):1050–1062, 2004 15612851

Morgenstern J, Blanchard KA, Morgan TJ, et al: Testing the effectiveness of cognitive-behavioral treatment for substance abuse in a community setting: within treatment and posttreatment findings. J Consult Clin Psychol 69(6):1007–1017, 2001a 11777104

Morgenstern J, Morgan TJ, McCrady BS, et al: Manual-guided cognitive-behavioral therapy training: a promising method for disseminating empirically supported substance abuse treatments to the practice community. Psychol Addict Behav 15(2):83–88, 2001b 11419234

Moyers TB, Martin T: Therapist influence on client language during motivational interviewing sessions. J Subst Abuse Treat 30(3):245–251, 2006 16616169

Moyers TB, Miller WR, Hendrickson SML: How does motivational interviewing work? Therapist interpersonal skill predicts client involvement within motivational interviewing sessions. J Consult Clin Psychol 73(4):590–598, 2005 16173846

Moyers TB, Martin T, Christopher PJ, et al: Client language as a mediator of motivational interviewing efficacy: where is the evidence? Alcohol Clin Exp Res 31(10 suppl):40s–47s, 2007 17880345

Peirce JM, Petry NM, Stitzer ML, et al: Effects of lower-cost incentives on stimulant abstinence in methadone maintenance treatment: a National Drug Abuse Treatment Clinical Trials Network study. Arch Gen Psychiatry 63(2):201–208, 2006 16461864

Petry NM, Peirce JM, Stitzer ML, et al: Effect of prize-based incentives on outcomes in stimulant abusers in outpatient psychosocial treatment programs: a national drug abuse treatment clinical trials network study. Arch Gen Psychiatry 62(10):1148–1156, 2005 16203960

Project MATCH Research Group: Matching Alcoholism Treatments to Client Heterogeneity: Project MATCH posttreatment drinking outcomes. J Stud Alcohol 58(1):7–29, 1997 8979210

Saunders B, Wilkinson C, Phillips M: The impact of a brief motivational intervention with opiate users attending a methadone programme. Addiction 90(3):415–424, 1995 7735025

Schwalbe CS, Oh HY, Zweben A: Sustaining motivational interviewing: a meta-analysis of training studies. Addiction 109(8):1287–1294, 2014 24661345

Sholomskas DE, Syracuse-Siewert G, Rounsaville BJ, et al: We don't train in vain: a dissemination trial of three strategies of training clinicians in cognitive-behavioral therapy. J Consult Clin Psychol 73(1):106–115, 2005 15709837

Smedslund G, Berg RC, Hammerstrøm KT, et al: Motivational interviewing for substance abuse. Cochrane Database Syst Rev (5):CD008063, 2011 21563163

Smith JL, Carpenter KM, Amrhein PC, et al: Training substance abuse clinicians in motivational interviewing using live supervision via teleconferencing. J Consult Clin Psychol 80(3):450–464, 2012 22506795

Swanson AJ, Pantalon MV, Cohen KR: Motivational interviewing and treatment adherence among psychiatric and dually diagnosed patients. J Nerv Ment Dis 187(10):630–635, 1999 10535657

Tross S, Campbell AN, Cohen LR, et al: Effectiveness of HIV/STD sexual risk reduction groups for women in substance abuse treatment programs: results of NIDA Clinical Trials Network Trial. J Acquir Immune Defic Syndr 48(5):581–589, 2008 18645513

Walters ST, Matson SA, Baer JS, et al: Effectiveness of workshop training for psychosocial addiction treatments: a systematic review. J Subst Abuse Treat 29(4):283–293, 2005 16311181

Weiss RD, Potter JS, Fiellin DA, et al: Adjunctive counseling during brief and extended buprenorphine-naloxone treatment for prescription opioid dependence: a 2-phase randomized controlled trial. Arch Gen Psychiatry 68(12):1238–1246, 2011 22065255

STUDENT REFLECTIONS

David L. Convissar, M.D.

Rutgers New Jersey Medical School 2016; Rutgers Anesthesiology 2020

As an internal medicine resident, I find that getting patients to make medical decisions that are in their best interest can be difficult, especially when involving addiction. The barriers that prevent the more educated, financially secure patients from making changes are the same ones that prevent those of lower socioeconomic standing and financial stability from making them as well. Be it the lack of knowledge of what will happen, the fear of failing, the fear of withdrawal, the list goes on. Working in hospitals and having experience with both populations, I've found myself having the exact same conversation with both a company CEO and a regular street junkie about their addictions. Techniques used in motivational interviewing (MI) are the commonality between the treatment of the two that facilitates change, because it comes from an inherent want, rather than from a financial advantage.

Cigarette smoking plagues both demographics and everyone in between, and having the conversation to quit is one I've had countless times, and will continue to have throughout my career. I've personally used tools from MI to try and get people to quit, be it partnering with the individual to create a team environment so that the individual knows he or she is not alone ("Lots of people have quit smoking"); being compassionate, to best understand the individual's situation and his or her addiction, despite not knowing myself what it's like ("Even though I've never been in your shoes, I imagine if must be very frightening"); or doing my best to evoke a personal strength in the individual to push him or her to know that he or she can do it ("You've gotten through harder things than this"). I've found that in real-life patient encounters, using these techniques has led to success.

Change is a step-by-step process, and even if the patient doesn't quit that day, it's gotten them thinking and placed them in the precontemplation, or even the contemplation, stage of change that leads to successful patient transformation.

Fundamentals of Motivational Interviewing

Caridad C. Ponce Martinez, M.D.

Bachaar Arnaout, M.D.

Steve Martino, Ph.D.

> The true mystery of the world is the visible, not the invisible.
>
> —*Oscar Wilde*

> You have brains in your head. You have feet in your shoes. You can steer yourself any direction you choose.
>
> —*Dr. Seuss*

In this chapter, we explore the fundamentals of motivation and change, first by presenting prior commonly held views about motivation and change in addictions treatment, then by describing *motivational interviewing* (MI), and finally by examining what MI and other psychotherapies have in common. We end with suggestions for teaching and supervision.

No discussion of MI would be adequate without first exploring motivation and change as part of treatment. Three elements of motivation have been identified: *direction* (what a person is trying to do), *effort* (how hard a person is trying), and *persistence* (how long a person keeps on trying) (Arnold et al. 2010). Abraham Maslow described the need for self-actualization, the desire to fulfill one's potential, as an important source for motivation (Maslow 1954)—a catalyst for change. Yet the predominant past view of substance users had been that patients with alcohol and drug addiction were inherently incapable of changing because of their rigid defensiveness in recognizing their problems, most embodied in the notion of their "denial" of addiction. In other words, substance users were "unmotivated" for change. The view of motivation as a personality trait rather than a state created a particular role for the clinician—one that justified the use of aggressive confrontational tactics purporting to break down resistance or "bust" through denial, accelerate the process of "hitting bottom," and reshape the addict's personality (Miller and Rollnick 1991).

Over time these directly confrontational and authoritarian interventions have yielded to addiction treatments that are guided by more contemporary and humane models of how people with substance use disorders change. In particular, we have gained a better understanding of motivation as a malleable state that is influenced by time, situation, clinician style, clinician expectancies, and patient expectancies. If motivation is viewed as the result of an interaction, then a change in the interaction could generate a different response and a change in motivation.

An important aspect of change is *ambivalence*, namely, having "mixed feelings" about staying the same versus making a behavioral change. For physicians and providers in allied fields, ambivalence has traditionally been approached by adopting an "expert role" in interactions with patients. Clinicians provide patients with information, expert opinion, and advice so that the patients can make the logical decision. However, in health care this seemingly logical change in behavior often does not occur, leading to interactions that can be fraught with frustration on behalf of both parties—patients do not feel understood or heard, while clinicians feel that their patients are not willing to change. This is the case not only in substance use disorders but also in chronic (e.g., diabetes, obesity) and acute (e.g., taking antibiotics as prescribed during a bacterial infection) conditions. As described in more detail below, MI views ambivalence as "a normal step on the road to change" (Miller and Rollnick 2013, p. 157). Clinicians using MI explore and help resolve ambivalence in favor of change.

MOTIVATIONAL INTERVIEWING

Motivational interviewing, first detailed in William R. Miller's landmark paper (Miller 1983) and then in the three editions of Miller and Stephen Rollnick's book *Motivational Interviewing* (Miller and Rollnick 1991, 2002, 2013), is deeply grounded in humanistic psychology, especially Carl Rogers's client-centered therapy.

Miller and Rollnick propose that change is a natural and ubiquitous process that is intrinsic to each person and that may occur without any outside intervention (Ellingstad et al. 2006; Schachter 1982). MI seeks to hasten this natural change process by creating an interpersonal situation, wherein the patient can engage in a collaborative dialogue that supports behavioral change from the patient's perspective. Fundamentally, MI is not exactly a *method* or a "bag of tricks"—not something that can be done *to* someone—but rather something that is done *with* someone, a way to *be with* another person that increases the likelihood that person will consider and become more committed to change.

MI views ambivalence as a part of the process of change—it focuses on exploring and resolving ambivalence and utilizing an individual's strengths as a way to facilitate change in a form that is congruent with the person's own values. Collaboration in the interaction between the patient and the clinician is key. Such collaboration can be conceptualized as two people looking at the same issue, trying to gain a shared perspective and working toward an agreeable solution.

As a result of ambivalence, arguments in favor of the change and against it emerge as *self-talk*, described as *change talk* and *sustain talk*, respectively. Language is crucial to MI in that a person becomes more committed to a position he or she argues for. One of the important roles for the clinician, therefore, is to shift the language of the session to include more change talk, which can thus lead to behavior change. The clinician's effort to guide the conversation in this way is in stark contrast to the directing style that is often found in clinical interactions. In fact, the term *righting reflex* has been utilized to describe the desire to fix what is deemed to be missing or wrong with patients, which may elicit relatively greater sustain talk than change talk. Similarly, a purely patient-centered approach, where the clinician primarily follows the patient, may not lead to behavior change in that the clinician does not purposively evoke and help enhance the patient's specific motivations for change.

The Spirit of Motivational Interviewing

The delivery of MI is characterized by a "spirit," highlighting a context for the conversations that is based on partnership, acceptance, compassion, and evocation.

*   *Partnership* values the patient's own perspective, creating a collaboration between the clinician and the patient. Although the clinician can (and should) provide some guidance in the process, it is ultimately up to the patient to decide whether change will occur. Additionally, guidance is best provided when the clinician understands, respects, and values the patient's perspective. The clinician may share information about a particular condition or treatment. However, the patient makes the decision—often informed by a clinician's advice or opinion—about how to proceed.
*   *Acceptance* contains at least four aspects (*absolute worth, affirmation, autonomy support*, and *accurate empathy*). Even when disagreeing with or disapproving of a patient's behavior, the clinician can convey acceptance by valuing and respecting the patient for his or her intrinsic worth as a human being (absolute worth), by making an effort to understand the world from the patient's perspective (accurate empathy), by respecting the patient's right and ability to

make his or her own choices (autonomy support), and by searching for and recognizing the patient's strengths and efforts (affirmation).

- *Compassion*, or beneficence, is not an emotional experience for the clinician, but instead an action, whereby the clinician seeks what is in the best interest of the patient. Without this element, the other elements within the spirit of MI, as well as the other techniques, could be ill-used to manipulate patients toward the goals of clinicians or other external factors. For example, using MI to encourage a patient to participate in a clinical trial that the clinician is heading would represent a conflict of interest, in which the clinician's desire to increase enrollment may become more valued than the potential benefit to the patient.

- *Evocation* requires that the clinician believe that the potential for change exists in the patient. The clinician seeks to draw out the patient's thoughts and values that support change, rather than imposing those endorsed by the clinician. By eliciting a person's motivations and skills for change, lasting change is more likely to occur. The answer, or "fix," best emanates from the patient's intrinsic motivations for change.

The Processes of Motivational Interviewing

In the conversation toward change, MI utilizes four processes: engaging, focusing, evoking, and planning. These processes overlap and are not always sequential. Instead, they build on each other, and there is flexibility to return to a previous process prior to continuing the conversation about change.

Engaging

Engaging refers to establishing and building rapport and learning about the patient. This is a crucial process in MI and in any therapeutic intervention for change to occur. The clinician seeks to engage the patient immediately in a collaborative conversation, a critical juncture when the patient forms an opinion about whether the clinician is compassionate, trustworthy, and knowledgeable. It is important to note, however, that the process of engaging must be cultivated throughout treatment and forms the foundation of all MI processes. The clinician's use of MI-consistent behaviors, in contrast with MI-inconsistent ones (e.g., direct confrontation, unsolicited advice, warnings), builds engagement along the way.

One way to improve engagement is with the use of *open questions, affirmations, reflections,* and *summaries* (OARS). Open questions are ones that invite elaborate answers and broad perspectives. Affirmations serve to highlight what the patient has done well, whether it is the patient's change efforts or strengths or a way to reframe a behavior or characteristic that brings attention to its positive elements. Reflections can be simple, where the clinician repeats or rephrases what the patient said, or complex, where the clinician makes a best guess about what the patient means (paraphrasing) or might say next (completing the paragraph). This serves to clarify information for the clinician and patient. Summaries can be viewed as *mega-reflections*, where the clinician provides a collection of thoughts, ideas, or feelings, with the goal of offering a linkage to information provided in the present or past conversations, summarizing ambivalence, or transitioning to another topic.

Feeling stuck during engaging?

Try to ask less and reflect more to demonstrate understanding and convey empathy. Try using more complex reflections and consider reflecting the patient's affect to get to the heart of the matter. Consider missed opportunities to affirm the patient, which might build rapport. Finally, sufficiently summarize what the patient has conveyed during the early part of the interview. The patient's hearing his or her full experience reflected back may help the patient feel more fully understood and connected with you.

Focusing

The process of *focusing* involves developing a specific agenda, developing goals for behavioral change, and adding direction to the conversation. Even in settings where the clinician has a clear role (e.g., substance abuse counseling, diabetes education, suicide prevention counseling), the goal or direction of the conversation should not be assumed. For example, consider a scenario in which a patient is court-mandated to alcohol abuse treatment, and abstinence becomes the main agenda for the clinician. The patient repeatedly discusses the stressor of losing custody of her children and her treatment priority is regaining custody of them, without apparent insight—according to the clinician—of the role of her alcohol abuse in the process. If the clinician continues to focus solely on the importance of abstinence, the patient is likely to feel ignored, misunderstood, and perhaps disrespected, which would hurt engagement and make a convergence of these goals even less likely.

When there are several choices in direction, a clinician might use a process called *agenda mapping* to bring focus to the conversation. Agenda mapping can be done in a concrete manner—for example, by writing down potential behavior change targets on paper in separate blocks or circles and then deciding collaboratively on the priorities. Consistent with the spirit of MI, a partnership is maintained in identifying a direction, and the clinician supports how the patient wants to proceed.

Sometimes patients may be unclear about what to address, how problems are related to one another, and how to proceed. Patients may be genuinely confused about what they are experiencing, and this may make it difficult for the clinician to bring focus to the session. The challenge is for the clinician and the patient to develop a mutual understanding of the patient's story and then to formulate and articulate the patient's major concerns. In essence, the clinician and the patient try to understand together what is occurring and bring this picture into focus. Like a guide, the clinician points to possible paths to follow after making sense of the big picture and proceeds according to the patient's wishes. This more complex process of focusing has been termed *orienting*.

Let's reconsider the scenario provided above, of a patient being court-mandated to alcohol abuse treatment. Over several sessions, the patient shares her frustration regarding the visitation schedule imposed by the court system for her to see her children. Her family is not providing any support after her husband left her, and she has to work two jobs in order to keep her apartment. She reports anxiety and insomnia and says that alcohol helps alleviate both. When asked about her major concerns, she mentions anxiety, financial strain, and her custody problems but does not see these problems as related to one another or to her drinking. The clinician helps brings these concerns together into a narrative that makes sense to the patient, and helps highlight the contributing role of her excessive alcohol use to each of these problems. The patient doesn't feel that she can begin to cut down on her alcohol use until her panic attacks are under control, bringing into focus a direction for their work together.

Feeling stuck during focusing?

Consider whether focusing is premature. Spend more time understanding the patient's dilemmas and mapping out the key motivational issues. Also, use the patient as a consultant to move from the general to the specific. For example, a patient may present with a number of concerns. The direction taken to address these concerns is best obtained via an exchange of information between the clinician and the patient, whereby the patient shares his or her priorities, and the destination for the collaborative work emerges. The clinician asks the patient for feedback and adjusts the direction accordingly, in order to maintain the therapeutic relationship (Miller and Rollnick 2013). At times, it may also be helpful to provide information and advice, with permission, when a patient is unsure where to focus and the input of the clinician might help the patient's considerations.

Evoking

Once a direction has been identified via focusing, *evoking* is the process through which there is exploration and explicit elicitation of a person's motivation for specific change. The skillful clinician hones in on those aspects of ambivalence that favor change (i.e., increased change talk) and resolves arguments that disfavor change (i.e., reduced sustain talk), both of which are associated with and predictive of subsequent behavioral change (Amrhein et al. 2003; Magill et al. 2014; Miller and Rose 2009). Evocation emphasizes open questions, affirmations, reflections, and summaries that encourage elaboration about motivations for change and bring focus to the patient's change-supportive statements. It also may involve the use of different evocative strategies (Table 2–1) to help a patient recognize his or her motivations for change in a more structured way.

Recognizing different types of change talk is a critical skill for clinicians to master in MI. The mnemonic DARN CAT captures different categories of change talk:

- *Desire:* indicates a patient's own desire for change, which can be offered spontaneously by the patient or elicited by the clinician (e.g., "I wish I didn't feel so sick from the shakes every morning").
- *Ability:* indicates a patient's capacity for change, even if he or she is not yet ready or committed to changing a behavior (e.g., "I've quit drinking during my pregnancies").
- *Reasons:* explores why a patient is considering making a change (e.g., "If I quit smoking, my house wouldn't smell like an ashtray all the time").
- *Need:* explores a sense of urgency regarding a behavior change (e.g., "I've got to stop injecting heroin or I'll die from an overdose").
- *Commitment:* indicates that a patient is likely to take action toward change (e.g., "I'm never buying another pack of cigarettes").
- *Activation:* indicates that the patient, by using language such as "I am willing," is leaning toward change but is not yet committed to taking action (e.g., "I'm willing to stop buying my cigarettes in bulk at the store").
- *Taking steps:* indicates that the patient has already taken some actions toward change, however small, which further increase his or her commitment (e.g., "I threw away all the ashtrays at home so that I'd have to walk outside in order to smoke").

Recognizing the type of change talk helps the clinician maintain direction during the session. For example, if the patient has spoken about desire, reasons, and need for change but not ability, the clinician would explore what makes the patient feel able to change. Patients who provide sufficient evidence of desire, ability, reasons, and need for change are likely prepared to commit to change

TABLE 2–1. Sample evocative strategies

Using scaling rulers	An *importance ruler* uses an imaginary scale (0–10) to determine level of perceived importance of a behavior change.
	A *confidence ruler* uses an imaginary scale (0–10) to determine a patient's perceived self-efficacy in carrying out a behavioral change.
	For each ruler, once a number is selected, the clinician asks why not a lower number (i.e., "Why a 4 and not a 1?") in order to elicit change talk. The clinician can then ask what would help for that number to increase (i.e., "What would help for that number to go from a 4 to a 7?") in order to elicit further change talk. The clinician uses OARS (open questions, affirmations, reflections, summaries) to strengthen elicited change talk.
Exploring goals and values	The clinician explores a patient's important values and goals and then asks the patient to consider how they fit with his or her current behavior, which may highlight discrepancy and create motivation for change. The clinician also asks how the patient's values and goals would be affected if change were to occur.
Looking forward, back, or at extremes	The clinician asks the patient to look forward into the future and imagine how the patient's life would improve if the behavior change were to occur. The clinician also has the option to ask the patient to look back in time to a period of healthier functioning and contrast it with current circumstances.
Exploring strengths or past successes	The clinician explores the patient's strengths and past successes and asks the patient to consider how these strengths or skills used to achieve success might apply to handling the current situation. This discussion may help improve the patient's confidence.
Exchanging information	The clinician provides information with the patient's permission (either by asking for it or when the clinician is asked) in a way that emphasizes patient autonomy. The clinician supports the patient's autonomy by asking what the patient makes of the shared information. Another technique, called *elicit–provide–elicit*, may be used as a means to first explore what the patient already knows about a subject, which is followed by the clinician providing additional or corrective information and then asking the patient what he or she makes of it.

and then develop a change plan (activation of motivations) and begin to take steps to implement the plan.

A common occurrence during the evocation process is the emergence of patient "resistance" as an expression of ambivalence toward change. The term *resistance* in this context was initially used by Miller and Rollnick (1991) in their first book about MI to describe any movement the patient had away from change. Their 2013 textbook reconceptualized the term *resistance* as comprising two different but related concepts: sustain talk and discord (Miller and Rollnick 2013). With *sustain talk*, the patient makes arguments in favor of the status quo. These arguments generally reflect what has been beneficial about the behavior or what makes change difficult or undesirable. Sustain talk is not pathological, but rather an expression of realistic ambivalence that often requires acknowledgment or exploration by the clinician. In MI, helping patients consider their arguments against change in juxtaposition with their arguments for change is a way to help them resolve their ambivalence.

In the case of *discord* there is a disturbance in the relationship between the clinician and the patient that undermines the patient's engagement and the broader motivational enhancement process. Discord may have occurred if the patient perceived the clinician as being consistently nonempathic or MI-inconsistent in a way that was off-putting to the patient (e.g., telling the patient what to do). The patient may demonstrate discord by becoming defensive, argumentative, interruptive, or disengaged. In MI, the clinician can respond to discord by focusing on maintaining the therapeutic alliance and using more reflections. The reflections become strategic in that they allow for the patient to feel heard and understood and the clinician to adjust the direction or pace of the conversation when necessary. The primary goal is to restore the relationship; and much as in other human relationships, it may be helpful to apologize, to take a break from a sensitive issue, or to affirm the individual's autonomy (Miller and Rollnick 2013).

Feeling stuck during evoking?

Consider in what areas change talk has emerged and what other areas might require more understanding. Does changing behavior matter enough to the patient? Does the patient seem confident that he or she is able to change? Are there obstacles to change that require exploration and problem solving? Summarize the conversation and see what the patient might add to the story he or she has told thus far. Continue to use your OARS and reflect change talk. If the change talk is general, ask for specifics. For example, consider the case of a patient saying, "I need to become a good father." Exploring the patient's view of what a good father is and what he could do to emulate that ideal (e.g., changing his substance use) could strengthen the patient's change talk. By exploring the emerging change talk and evoking more of it, you help the patient talk himself into change.

Planning

At some point in the motivational process, a patient may show signs of readiness for change, as indicated by using more change talk and less sustain talk, asking questions about change, and envisioning what it would be like to make the change. When the clinician recognizes these signs, he or she should open up the *planning* process. Commonly, the clinician begins planning for change with the patient by collectively summarizing the patient's major change talk and then asking a key question that might evoke the patient's commitment to change (e.g., "So what do you think you will do at this point?"). If the patient indicates a change goal, then the clinician proceeds with a discussion of the patient's change plans. Recognize that ambivalence is normal at this stage and may emerge as the patient considers what he or she will do. If this occurs, the clinician reflects the patient's ambivalence and helps the patient resolve it before continuing with the planning process. In some cases, a patient will remain ambivalent within the session and will not make plans for change at that time.

Assuming there is sufficient engagement, a clear, shared goal, and sufficient commitment to initiate behavior change, the clinician develops a change plan with the patient (Table 2–2). The change plan typically consists of four major elements: setting clear goals, exploring options for change, deciding on a plan, and committing to the plan. Envision a situation where a patient tells the clinician that he is thinking about cutting back on his marijuana use and has recently stopped smoking in the mornings before work. The clinician "tests the water" by asking the patient if he is ready to talk about how he may go about doing this. The clinician recapitulates the change talk offered by the patient—he needs to be more focused at work because his boss has noticed some mistakes recently, he wants to spend more quality time with his children, and he has already started by deleting the telephone number of one of his two dealers. The patient reiterates his desire to stop smoking marijuana. They explore ways that the patient has reduced his smoking in the past, as options to help him stop at this time—he could take on a new project at work, sign up to be a softball assistant coach for his son's team, or enlist his wife's help in not bringing marijuana into the house. Given that the patient's main motivation is to provide a good example for his children, together the patient and clinician decide that the patient will sign up as a softball assistant coach. He will share his plan with his wife, begin to practice softball with his son in the afternoons when he may wish to otherwise smoke, and meet with the clinician again in one week to find out how the plan is working. The clinician strengthens the patient's commitment to the plan by writing down the steps that

TABLE 2–2.	Key elements of a change plan
Setting clear goals	The clinician helps the patient set clear goals for behavior change.
Exploring options for change	The clinician helps the patient identify ways to achieve the goals in the context of the patient's preferences, values, and strengths. The aim is to establish options, not critique them.
Deciding on a plan	The clinician and patient come to a shared agreement about which options the patient will exercise and further refine them, including anticipating obstacles to change, markers of progress, and social supports to be accessed as needed.
Committing to the plan	Once a plan is developed, the clinician helps strengthen the patient's commitment to carrying out this plan by asking for a commitment to it, summarizing the steps, and affirming steps the patient may have already taken to initiate change.

the patient has described, and affirms the patient in his decision to delete his marijuana dealer's telephone number.

Feeling stuck during planning?

Consider whether planning is premature. If developing a plan is difficult, consider whether 1) there is not a clear shared goal, 2) the patient is insufficiently involved in the change planning discussion, 3) as an "expert," you're coming up with the solution or are prescribing what the patient should do, or 4) more motivational enhancement is necessary.

MOTIVATIONAL INTERVIEWING AND OTHER PSYCHOTHERAPIES

MI targets behavior but does not do so by providing models, skills, or solutions. MI is often delivered as a brief intervention, which has been shown to have at least modest successful results after only a few sessions (Lundahl et al. 2010). It is compatible with other treatment approaches, and this allows its integration into many types of clinical practices and providers. In multiple studies, these combinations have included MI in addition to feedback, education, self-help manuals, cognitive-behavioral therapy (CBT), skills training, 12-step groups, and stress management (Arkowitz and Miller 2008; Baer et al. 1999).

As noted in the preface to this book, the objective is to provide a practical text written for clinicians by clinicians. All of the authors of the book's chapters are seasoned addiction clinicians with different roles and theoretical backgrounds—some with a cognitive-behavioral background, others with a passion for psychodynamics or motivational interventions, and many with an avid interest in psychopharmacology. What unites them despite the theoretical differences is the ability to work with individuals toward behavioral change and to write about the terrain they have explored during such journeys. Not uncommonly, advocates of different theoretical approaches strive to refute one another or point out the deficiencies of theoretical perspectives other than their own. In line with the gentle and nonjudgmental approach of humanistic psychology, we wish to do quite the opposite: to point out what MI has in common with other psychotherapies, which together form the rich and fascinating mosaic of the psychotherapeutic community.

The therapeutic relationship may be the most central element to all effective psychotherapies. The therapist's empathy for, attunement with, and acceptance of the patient enable the therapeutic dialogue to unfold and the exploration of challenging details about the person's life and goals to occur. This "empowerment through acceptance" can be viewed as essential to all successful psychotherapy and to change in general. As noted earlier, change can be viewed as natural and intrinsic to each person and is facilitated in psychotherapy by creating a supportive and accepting environment.

This dialectic of acceptance and change is most clearly stated in the serenity prayer and 12-step literature, and is perhaps even more typically associated with *dialectical behavior therapy,* or DBT. It is worth noting that acceptance does not mean indifference; rather, it is a way to slow down and take note of what is in one's mind. The confidence that acceptance brings gives the person the time to think and decide whether and how to respond to an impulse, rather than equating impulse with behavior. This ability to uncouple impulse from behavior is, in turn, a central component in CBT.

In psychodynamics, commonalities with MI and humanistic psychology may be especially prominent in the interpersonal, relational, and intersubjective traditions. Psychodynamic work is often portrayed as a balancing of supportive (i.e., accepting) and expressive (i.e., challenging) components, well embodied by the words "I do enough psychotherapy (often seen as more supportive) to make psychoanalysis (often seen as more challenging) possible" (Stefan R. Zicht, personal communication, 2007). As disputable as the distinctions between psychoanalytic terms may be, this mental space that enables dialogue and makes change possible has been referred to differently by many authors, variously described as "transitional space" (Winnicott 1971), "negotiation" (Pizer 1998), and "thirdness" (Benjamin 2004), among others.

It is in this environment that the will of the individual is reified, empowering him or her to change. Empowering constitutes the opposite of what is often called *enabling*. Enabling creates an atmosphere in which another dialectic—of dominance and dependence, of clinging and discarding, of push-pull relationships—fuels current patterns and hampers change.

Miller and Rollnick (1991, 2002, 2013) consider MI to be consistent with other psychotherapeutic modalities. They also note that MI can be used in practice as part of an alternation model, particularly when motivation for change becomes the challenge at any point in treatment, with other modalities used for other tasks. Alternatively, MI may become part of a clinician's style, in which the processes of engaging, focusing, evoking, and planning are used within a model integrated with other treatment modalities. A related aspect of the integrative model is the incorporation of the spirit of MI into practice, regardless of the specific psychotherapeutic modality used, so that interactions with patients are based on partnership, acceptance, compassion, and evocation.

Some of MI's most enduring treatment effects have been found when it has been used as a prelude to more intensive standard treatment programs (Lundahl and Burke 2009). This has been applied in clinical practice, where blends of MI with other psychotherapeutic modalities such as CBT and 12-step facilitation are often used. In particular, MI and CBT are often seen as complementary, with the former focusing on the *why* and the latter addressing the *how* of change (Carroll 1998). In research this has been applied in the COMBINE Study, in which components of MI, CBT, and 12-step facilitation, as well as support system involvement targeting alcohol dependence, were blended into a combined behavioral intervention (Anton et al. 2006).

SUGGESTIONS FOR TEACHING AND SUPERVISION

Teaching MI can be a very gratifying experience. The difficulty, however, often lies in MI being a "methodless" method that places an emphasis on spirit and attitude before technique. While the theory and technique of MI can be fairly easily grasped in intellectual terms, the shift in attitude and practice that MI welcomes is a lengthier process.

The medical profession trains its students to gather extensive histories with focused and detailed accounts of patients' complaints and symptoms. Not infrequently, students shower patients with a litany of closed-ended questions and find it difficult to ask open questions and to then follow them with reflections. Another difficulty is the illusion that the clinician can, and in fact *has to*, change patients by convincing them and giving extensive expert advice. Perhaps the high stress and expectations inherent in the medical profession are often dealt with through a need to control, especially among junior physicians and medical students. While there certainly is a place for closed-ended questions, gathering detailed data, and assured expert advice and recommendations, it is valuable in effecting eventual behavior change to encourage students to try to adopt the spirit of collaboration, evocation, and autonomy that MI invites.

This shift in attitude is likely better taught by demonstration, wherein the teaching itself is conducted in this spirit. After explaining the basic tenets of MI, the teacher engages the students in a discussion in the spirit of MI, embodied by using open questions, affirmations, reflections, and summaries (OARS) as teaching tools, and empowering students by accepting their views even when they differ from the teacher's views. Modeling can be followed by the teacher and student participating in a role-play to practice the skills. By practicing MI, the students can internalize its spirit (Miller and Rollnick 2013; Rosengren 2009).

A key aspect of teaching MI is having students learn it using experiential activities that sequentially build their skills over time. Miller and Moyers (2006) have described eight stages and associated skills by which clinicians become increasingly proficient. Training begins with helping clinicians become open to the assumptions and principles of MI and grasping the MI spirit as a style of interacting with patients, particularly developing accurate empathy (stage 1). Training then moves toward teaching and honing clinician patient-centered counseling skills (stage 2). Next, clinicians learn to recognize, elicit, and reinforce change talk, particularly identifying commitment language (stages 3 and 4) and handling resistance skillfully (stage 5). Shifting to change planning and strengthening commitment to change follows (stages 6 and 7). Finally, with MI skills solidified, clinicians learn how to flexibly shift back and forth from MI to other approaches (stage 8). David Rosengren, an experienced clinician and MI trainer, has summarized his training into a 5-step format: tell (didactic or exercise to elicit information), see (the skill in action), do in slow motion (individual or group exercise), perform (the skill in real time), and build (on increasing complexity and number of skills). His book *Building Motivational Interviewing Skills: A Practitioner Workbook* (Rosengren 2009) is an excellent resource for these types of training activities.

Eventually students need to conduct MI with real patients and require supervision, where the interaction between the patient and the supervisee is paralleled by the interaction between supervisee and supervisor. Taping sessions after gaining the patient's consent offers a more fine-grained account of the session and can be very beneficial to master the therapy. This type of direct observation of the student's session is critical in that therapists learning MI have been shown to overestimate their abilities (Martino et al. 2009). Moreover, supervisors can rate the students' MI skills, using established rating systems (Martino et al.

2008; Moyers et al. 2016) that can then provide the basis for offering students feedback and coaching. The combination of repeated direct observation, feedback, and coaching following didactic/workshop training has been the only method to date that has been shown to significantly develop clinicians' skills in MI (Miller et al. 2004). Rosengren (2009) likens practicing MI without receiving feedback to hitting golf balls in the dark: "one may know how the swing feels, but there is no information about what happened and what adjustments need to be made" (p. 2).

Making this process collaborative and positive rather than solely supervisor driven is important. One of the authors' (B.A.) previous supervisors encourages students' self-evaluation during supervision, where the student is asked to provide three skills that were performed well during the therapeutic session with the patient, and then balance them with providing one area in which the student feels he or she needs improvement. Students are often amused by this ratio of 3:1, and at times they are more ready to engage in self-criticism rather than find what skills they have actually mastered.

An often-voiced concern among teachers is that some students are "natural" motivational interviewers while others are not. In our experience, it is valuable to always draw on the positive and affirm students wherever they may be on their learning journey. Overall, good teachers and supervisors are able to roll with the students' resistances and certainly avoid arguing and attempting to convince the students to drop reservations they have about MI.

Finally, it is often helpful to use a clear and concise table that summarizes MI and can be used as a flashcard during role-play exercises. We provide an example in Figure 2–1.

KEY POINTS

- Change is natural and intrinsic and can be hastened by a supportive yet directive approach.

- Motivational interviewing (MI) is an approach for developing the patient's intrinsic motivation for behavior change by using a style of communication that blends patient-centered listening skills with methods directed at eliciting the patient's motivation and commitment for change.

- The clinician adopts a spirit of interacting with the patient, marked by partnership, acceptance, compassion, and evocation of the patient's resources and motivations for change.

- MI happens in four overlapping processes that build on one another: engaging, focusing, evoking, and planning.

Motivational Interviewing		
Spirit (PACE)	Processes (EFEP)	Motivational interviewing in four steps
Partnership	Engaging	1. OARS: Ask Open Questions Affirm Reflect Summarize
Acceptance	Focusing	2. Focus (general → specific) May start to give I & A (Information and Advice)
Compassion	Evoking	3. Elicit change talk Consider using two rulers: • Importance ruler • Confidence ruler Follow each ruler with two questions: • Why x and not x – 3? • What would it take to go from x to x + 3?
Evocation	Planning	4. Negotiate a plan (general → specific)

FIGURE 2–1. **Example of flashcard summarizing motivational interviewing that can be used during role-play exercises.**

- MI core skills include use of fundamental patient-centered listening skills known as OARS (open questions, affirmations, reflections, and summaries) and giving information and advice in an MI-consistent manner.

- The clinician's ability to recognize and elicit change talk in the context of the spirit of the approach is the main mechanism by which MI is presumed to work.

- MI has many parallels with other modes of therapy, and the ability to provide change-oriented therapy is seen as common to many schools of psychotherapy.

- Teaching and supervision are effectively done in a supportive and collaborative manner that is consistent with the spirit of MI. Skills can be mastered and applied with adequate instruction and supervision. Change in trainees is natural.

STUDY QUESTIONS

1. Motivational interviewing (MI) is most closely related to

   A. Psychoanalysis.
   B. Behaviorism.
   C. Humanistic psychology.
   D. The 12-step tradition.

2. The spirit of MI lies in

   A. Criticism, elucidation, diagnosis, and analysis.
   B. Creativity, expansion, passivity, and advocacy.
   C. Confrontation, criticism, education, and authority.
   D. Partnership, acceptance, compassion, and evocation.

3. Which of the following patient statements best predicts his or her readiness and commitment to change?

   A. "If I don't stop drinking, my liver cirrhosis will only get worse."
   B. "Last week I began leaving my cigarettes in the trunk of my car while driving so I wouldn't be tempted to smoke."
   C. "I could go for a walk after dinner instead of smoking a cigarette."
   D. "I desperately want to be able to fall asleep without needing a marijuana joint."

4. MI often can be successfully combined with other therapeutic modalities. This statement is

   A. False, because any association with other therapies will confuse the patient.
   B. True, because MI is compatible with many approaches.
   C. Dangerous, because therapists should always be passionate advocates of only one psychotherapeutic school.
   D. Irrelevant, because competent therapists spontaneously know what to do without the need to learn MI.

5. Teaching and supervision of MI

    A. Are best done in an accepting and collaborative manner.

    B. Are best done through confrontation to emphasize contrast with the style of MI.

    C. Require that the student undergo his or her own motivational therapy.

    D. Should focus on convincing the student that MI is better than other therapies.

REFERENCES

Amrhein PC, Miller WR, Yahne CE, et al: Client commitment language during motivational interviewing predicts drug use outcomes. J Consult Clin Psychol 71(5):862–878, 2003 14516235

Anton RF, O'Malley SS, Ciraulo DA, et al: Combined pharmacotherapies and behavioral interventions for alcohol dependence: the COMBINE study: a randomized controlled trial. JAMA 295(17):2003–2017, 2006 16670409

Arkowitz H, Miller WR: Learning, applying, and extending motivational interviewing, in Motivational Interviewing in the Treatment of Psychological Problems. Edited by Arkowiz H, Westra HA, Miller WR, et al. New York, Guilford, 2008, pp 1–25

Arnold J, Randall R, Patterson F, et al: Work Psychology: Understanding Human Behaviour in the Workplace, 5th Edition. Don Mills, Ontario, Canada, Pearson Education, 2010

Baer JS, Kivlahan DR, Donovan DM: Integrating skills training and motivational therapies. Implications for the treatment of substance dependence. J Subst Abuse Treat 17(1–2):15–23, 1999 10435249

Benjamin J: Beyond doer and done to: an intersubjective view of thirdness. Psychoanal Q 73(1):5–46, 2004 14750464

Carroll KM: A Cognitive-Behavioral Approach: Treating Cocaine Addiction. Therapy Manuals for Drug Abuse, Manual 1. NIH Publ No 98-4308. Rockville, MD, National Institute on Drug Abuse, April 1998

Ellingstad TP, Sobell LC, Sobell MB, et al: Self-change: A pathway to cannabis abuse resolution. Addict Behav 31(3):519–530, 2006 15967588

Lundahl B, Burke BL: The effectiveness and applicability of motivational interviewing: a practice-friendly review of four meta-analyses. J Clin Psychol 65(11):1232–1245, 2009 19739205

Lundahl BW, Kunz C, Brownell C, et al: A meta-analysis of motivational interviewing: twenty-five years of empirical studies. Res Soc Work Pract 20(2):137–160, 2010

Magill M, Gaume J, Apodaca TR, et al: The technical hypothesis of motivational interviewing: a meta-analysis of MI's key causal model. J Consult Clin Psychol 82(6):973–983, 2014 24841862

Martino S, Ball SA, Nich C, et al: Community program therapist adherence and competence in motivational enhancement therapy. Drug Alcohol Depend 96(1–2):37–48, 2008 18328638

Martino S, Ball S, Nich C, et al: Correspondence of motivational enhancement treatment integrity ratings among therapists, supervisors, and observers. Psychother Res 19(2):181–193, 2009 19396649

Maslow AH: Motivation and Personality. New York, Harper & Row, 1954

Miller WR: Motivational interviewing with problem drinkers. Behavioural Psychotherapy 11(2):147–172, 1983

Miller WR, Moyers TB: Eight stages in learning motivational interviewing. Journal of Teaching in the Addictions 5(1):3–17, 2006

Miller WR, Rollnick S: Motivational Interviewing: Preparing People for Change. New York, Guilford, 1991

Miller WR, Rollnick S: Motivational Interviewing: Preparing People for Change, 2nd Edition. New York, Guilford, 2002

Miller WR, Rollnick S: Motivational Interviewing: Helping People Change, 3rd Edition. New York, Guilford, 2013

Miller WR, Rose GS: Toward a theory of motivational interviewing. Am Psychol 64(6):527–537, 2009 19739882

Miller WR, Yahne CE, Moyers TB, et al: A randomized trial of methods to help clinicians learn motivational interviewing. J Consult Clin Psychol 72(6):1050–1062, 2004 15612851

Moyers TB, Rowell LN, Manuel JK, et al: The Motivational Interviewing Treatment Integrity Code (MITI 4): Rationale, Preliminary Reliability and Validity. J Subst Abuse Treat 65:36–42, 2016 26874558

Pizer SA: Building Bridges: The Negotiation of Paradox in Psychoanalysis. Hillsdale, NJ, Analytic Press, 1998

Rosengren DB: Building Motivational Interviewing Skills: A Practitioner Workbook. New York, Guilford, 2009

Schachter S: Recidivism and self-cure of smoking and obesity. Am Psychol 37(4):436–444, 1982 7103240

Winnicott DW: The use of an object and relating through identifications, in Playing and Reality. London, Psychology Press, 1971, pp 86–94

STUDENT REFLECTIONS

Isaac Johnson
Yale School of Medicine, MS2

Several things struck me when I read this chapter. How often have we heard that a patient is "unmotivated" or in "denial," when the techniques we sometimes use are the very tactics that could make a patient feel marginalized or misunderstood, driving the patient to maintain the status quo? This chapter describes motivation as a state rather than a trait. It views patient motivation as something that I, as a medical student, have the capacity to impact by working alongside a patient, rather than adopting the "expert role." I find this perspective very useful, and I'll remember it when I talk with patients. This chapter also reinforced for me the notion that exploring a patient's ambivalence about change is important in order for the patient to feel respected and to help the patient move toward change. I was reminded that the patient makes the decision to change, not the clinician, and that my job is to help the patient find his or her own desire for change. I must respect the timing and pace of that change.

The authors advise us to "try to ask less and reflect more" what the patient is saying about his or her values and desires, readiness to change, and ambivalence about change. I love the question that the authors recommend asking to help the patient move toward commitment: "So what do you think you will do at this point?" I can see myself applying this method in many clinical encounters. This chapter recommends that students "adopt the spirit of collaboration, evocation, and autonomy." I feel motivated to incorporate these principles into my clinical practice.

What I learned most from this chapter is the importance of having an attitude of respect, rather than judgment, for the patient's process and choices. I found many of the techniques and concepts in this chapter to be relevant to any clinical interaction, whether the chief concern is substance misuse or not. The skills I learned in this chapter will allow me to build on the patient-centered skills I've already developed in order to more fully cultivate the patient's potential to be his or her own best advocate.

▶Chapter

3

Engaging

Teofilo E. Matos Santana, M.D.
Ayana Jordan, M.D., Ph.D.

> In my early professional years I was asking the question: How can I
> treat, or cure, or change this person? Now I would phrase the question
> in this way: How can I provide a relationship, which this person may
> use for his own personal growth?
>
> —*Carl Rogers*

Engagement is the first step in the therapeutic relationship and constitutes the foundation of motivational interviewing (MI) work. It is the process by which the patient and clinician agree to connect, to disclose, and to work together comfortably. The engaging process is variable and dynamic; sometimes the process occurs early, with relative ease, while at other times it requires effort from both the clinician and the patient. Many factors can influence the strength of the relationship and the pace at which engagement happens. The thoughts and feelings a clinician or a patient may have during the encounter can and will affect engagement. For example, diverse experiences and vulnerabilities the patient and clinician possess can affect the engaging process. In this way, engaging is a two-way process. To promote patient collaboration, the clinician should be aware of these factors and work proactively to provide an environment where the patient feels safe to share information.

A well-engaged patient will participate in the complex process of change, verbalizing fears and barriers preventing change, while also communicating values and thoughts congruent with change. Revisiting the engagement process throughout MI helps to solidify the relational foundation of this therapeutic modality. Investing time in a genuine engagement will result in a more satisfactory therapeutic relationship and promote adherence and retention in treatment. People who are actively engaged are more likely to fully participate and benefit from treatment (Fuertes et al. 2007). In this chapter we delineate the goals of engaging, communication styles that support engagement, and ways in which engaging affects therapeutic outcomes. We then discuss the core MI communication skills, known as OARS (open questions, affirmations, reflections, and summaries), and provide examples of their use in clinical practice.

GOALS OF ENGAGING

Given the importance of engaging in MI, it is necessary to understand the basic goals of engagement:

* Ensure the patient participates in treatment.
* Help the patient feel safe to share information.
* Allow the patient to feel understood, respected, and trusted.
* Allow participation in a collaborative way.

When these goals are met, the patient is willing to explore the process of behavioral change and is more likely to engage in the other processes of MI. There are positive actions that can enhance and facilitate change, whereas certain modes of communication or traps may promote disengagement. In the next two sections, we examine some of these factors in greater detail.

COMMUNICATION STYLES IN THE ENGAGEMENT PROCESS

Nonverbal Communication

Nonverbal communication can affect interpersonal interaction. A receptive, flexible, and curious attitude is encouraged. An engaging clinician is present and responsive, with good eye contact and reactive facial expressions sensitive to the matter of discussion.

According to Miller and Rollnick (2013), some nonverbal, concrete behaviors that promote engagement are

* Practicing good listening.
* Providing undivided attention.
* Comforting with eye contact and genuine facial expression.

These actions can signal to the patient that the clinician cares about him or her and is genuinely invested in helping. These three behaviors are consistent with good nonverbal listening. A clinician who keeps comfortable eye contact, avoids getting distracted by looking at the chart or at the clock, and is able to mirror the patient's emotions, while responding through facial expressions, is working to engage the patient in the process of change.

Verbal Communication

There are other ways to reinforce a healthy engagement by thoughtfully choosing words during the interview process and employing reflective listening. In this subsection we describe how the interview is used as an aid for engagement, explain reflective listening as a tool in the interview process, and highlight how in a good interview reflective listening is used to facilitate engagement.

The Interview as an Aid for Engagement

The interview provides the necessary structure for the clinician's evaluation and treatment of a patient's health needs. The clinician in the clinical interview not only has the goal of obtaining and transmitting accurate information, but also strives to engage the patient in a way that promotes a safe environment. The most consistent factor predicting therapeutic gain in the healing of medical and psychological conditions is the quality of the therapeutic relationship and the patient's pretreatment personality dimensions (Blatt and Zuroff 2005). Personalization of the interview and the adoption of a conscious attitude toward the patient's individual needs will facilitate engagement.

The way information is gathered during the interview can have an impact on the engagement process. Balancing the amount of questions asked, applying nonverbal skills, and having the goals of engaging in mind can all help to promote engagement. In addition to nonverbal communication, a useful tool that can be utilized throughout the interview is reflective listening.

Reflective Listening

Reflective listening is the process by which the clinician listens carefully to the patient and makes an informed guess about what the patient means or is trying to communicate. A reflective comment should be provided as a statement, rather than a question: "You may not be ready to quit smoking cannabis." Reflective listening can help the patient feel heard and allows the clinician to demonstrate if he or she has a good understanding of what the patient is communicating. Usually, if the reflective statement is correct, the patient feels affirmed, thereby increasing the strength of the engagement. Reflections can be used in all four processes of MI, starting with engagement.

Reflective listening helps the clinician to join with the patient collaboratively in the conversation. A good reflection should encourage the patient's continued self-exploration and constitutes a valuable tool in the clinical interview. The concept of reflection as a tool of engagement will be discussed in greater detail later in the chapter.

ACTIONS THAT INTERFERE WITH ENGAGEMENT

There are actions that can be damaging to the engagement process. Miller and Rollnick (2013) describe these behaviors as "traps that promote disengagement." Some of these traps include

- Using excessive questioning that would place the patient in a passive role.
- Adopting a domineering expert role, where both parties are set up for an uneven power relationship.
- Prematurely focusing on and labeling a patient's problems and goals for change, without engaging in a collaborative relationship.
- Judging and blaming the patient, which only increases resistance to change.
- Informally chatting, without talking about salient clinical issues.

The "traps of disengagement" can risk, weaken, or threaten the therapeutic engagement and can affect the next processes of MI.

ENGAGING AT THE CORE OF THE THERAPEUTIC RELATIONSHIP

Multiple studies have shown that the therapeutic relationship is easily the most important ingredient in any therapeutic modality (Crits-Christoph et al. 2011; Farrell et al. 2009; Karver et al. 2006), and MI is not an exception. The therapeutic relationship is a partnership or collaborative process between the patient and clinician in the common fight to overcome suffering and self-destructive behavior (Bordin 1979). The therapeutic relationship consists of three main elements: 1) agreement on the goals or targets of treatment, 2) agreement on the tasks or behaviors to achieve the defined goals, and 3) the development of a personal bond between patient and clinician, made up of reciprocal feelings (Bordin 1979). Engaging, if done correctly, is at the core of this therapeutic relationship and strengthens the dynamic by promoting collaboration in treatment. Engaging allows patients to feel safe, heard, and respected. It is difficult to imagine a therapeutic relationship formed in the absence of an engagement process.

ROLE OF ENGAGING IN IMPROVING OUTCOMES

There is a proven, linear relationship between the quality of the therapeutic interaction and treatment outcomes (Martin et al. 2000). The patient's experience of the engagement process, early in treatment, is significantly related to the degree of symptom reduction (Blatt and Zuroff 2005). The goal of a beneficial engagement should aim to reduce vulnerability to distress and allow a patient to develop adaptive capacities to the challenges of daily life (Blatt and Zuroff 2005).

In the search for an active component in the engagement process, it has been found that certain therapeutic relationship variables are more strongly related to positive outcomes than others (Karver et al. 2006). For example, in the youth population, where it can be challenging to foster behavioral change, relationship variables such as a clinician's interpersonal skills, a parent's willingness to participate in treatment, the youth's willingness to participate in treatment, affect toward the therapist, and the therapeutic relationship itself were found to influence treatment outcomes (Karver et al. 2006). These components were all proven to be vital for a clinician who strives to guide a patient through the complex process of change. Clinician self-disclosure was not associated with better outcomes. Therefore, a patient-centered approach, as implemented by an MI-spirited clinician, not only establishes a comfortable interaction but also results in better treatment outcomes. Engaging provides the "motor" or energy necessary to promote and maintain a strong therapeutic relationship.

CORE COMMUNICATION SKILLS IN MOTIVATIONAL INTERVIEWING: OARS

Open questions, Affirmations, Reflections, and Summaries, collectively known as OARS, are the core, foundational skills in engaging, and they are also the core skills used throughout the remaining three processes of MI. Taking into account the factors that facilitate engagement, including good nonverbal and verbal communication, while being sure to avoid the "traps of disengagement," we can now review the core communication skills in MI.

Open Questions

Open questions prompt patients to explore, freely think, and express themselves. An open question should produce information without leading someone to a specific answer. It enhances patient autonomy and allows patients to say what is important to them, according to their priorities. On the contrary, closed questions can lead patients to a specific answer that may hamper the process of open exploration. Provided below are ways to ask about similar concepts, using both open and closed questions.

Open Questions

- How has it been for you since we last met?
- What struggles have you had?

- How has drinking affected you?
- What gets in the way of your sobriety plans?
- How has this behavior affected your life?
- How important is it to include your family in your life?

Closed Questions

- Did you relapse?
- How many drinks did you have?
- Why can't you stay sober? Is it because you can't resist temptation?
- Alcohol has affected your life in so many ways. Can you tell me one?
- Isn't how you are affecting your family, important for you?

The last questions not only are closed but also are distant from the MI spirit. These questions do not promote engaging. The closed question "How many drinks did you have?" requires estimation of a quantity "I had 5 drinks," thereby providing a fact, rather than an understanding of the patient. The last three closed questions not only are limiting but also have a judgmental, labeling, and paternalistic tone, which rarely helps engage patients in the process of change.

Affirming

Affirmations are used to genuinely highlight the strengths of the patient while also promoting self-efficacy. Patients who come for assistance in the process of change have often been exposed to criticism and may be expecting people to point out their flaws and mistakes. By affirming, the clinician acknowledges that despite struggles and negative habits, people also have positive aspects in their intention and behavior. Affirmations allow patients to feel valued and respected by reinforcing the patient's positive attributes. Change is often difficult because people are generally ambivalent about their behaviors, so emphasizing a patient's positive skill or trait can help stimulate change. Sometimes negative behaviors have become so recurrent and pervasive that patients have forgotten about the other side, the side that desires change. This side may be more congruent with their inner values and beliefs. By acknowledging their strengths, the goal of affirming is for patients to feel valued and also to encourage continued participation in treatment.

Affirmations can also be used to promote self-efficacy by emphasizing past successes or positive traits. Throughout the patient encounter, one should be looking for strengths, past successes in behavioral change, and good efforts to reinforce a patient's ability to carry out their own stated goals. For example, in the case of patients with substance use disorders, past sobriety time or significant reduction of use are good ways to affirm the patient's behavior. Many times patients will spontaneously offer historical information about strengths and successes. The clinician can use this information to affirm the patient and focus on constructive behavior. Affirmations are a way to help patients see themselves as valuable, useful, ready, and capable of change.

Effective affirmations are genuine and strive to be accurate. Affirmations will not be useful if the patient notices a lack of truth or superficiality in an affirming statement. It is usually not difficult to find positive qualities and strengths in every patient. Positive attributes and strengths can be gathered by using open questions. If a clinician is having trouble appreciating a strength for a particular patient, this may be a good time to revisit the MI spirit. The clinician should make sure to adopt a nonjudgmental, respectful tone, always defending the patient's autonomy, while striving for collaboration and partnership. Affirmations will increase the level of engagement by balancing the relationship and decreasing any discord.

Affirmative Statements

- It is great that you continue to think of ways to be a better father.
- You continue to search for a job, and that's no small thing.
- Even when you continue drinking, you still make it in for your appointments.
- While you continue using cocaine, you were able to cut down on your use considerably.

Reflecting

Reflections are one of the most important elements of MI. Miller and Rollnick (2013) refer to a reflection as "a reasonable guess as to what the original meaning was, and gives a voice to this guess in the form of a statement." Often considered "the thing to do when you have no idea what to do," a reflection is a valuable tool in understanding the patient, and it is a key component of active listening. *Reflective listening* is a combination of open questions plus reflections, which help patients engage while allowing the clinician to gather accurate information. In the process of communication, sometimes words are articulated in a manner that is congruent with a thought or intention, but sometimes the two are incongruent, and the patient doesn't mean what was just said. When a clinician offers a reflection or uses reflective listening, the patient has a chance to examine what was said and verify if it is indeed congruent with what he or she is thinking and with his or her intention.

Features of a Good Reflection

The reflection from the clinician should be voiced as a statement rather than a question (Table 3–1). In this way, the clinician is neither intrusive nor demanding. The reflection serves as an invitation to explore further, clarify, or confirm the guess. This mode of communication helps with engaging, allowing the clinician to obtain accurate knowledge, make fewer assumptions, and establish congruency with the patient. The reflections should be close to the patient's expressed ideas, without deviating too much from the flow of what's been communicated. A good reflection does not interfere with the idea being conveyed, but rather enhances the idea. If the clinician makes an inaccurate guess, a well-engaged patient will provide clarification and continue with the natural flow of the conversation.

TABLE 3–1.   Features of a good reflection

A good reflection . . .

   is framed as a statement rather than a question.

   takes the form of a statement that stays close to the patient's idea.

   promotes self-exploration.

   is concise, direct, and easy to understand.

   does not block the flow of information the patient is verbalizing.

   enhances the patient's idea while staying close to the subject of discussion.

Types of Reflections

There are two basic types of reflections, simple and complex. Definitions and examples of these two reflections are outlined in greater detail below.

Simple reflections

This type of reflection often involves repetition of words, with the clinician adding very little or nothing to what the patient has stated. Simple reflections can help the flow of conversation, used to acknowledge or highlight the importance of what has been said. Examples of some simple reflections are as follows:

> PATIENT: I'm fed up with this cocaine use.
> CLINICIAN 1: You are fed up with your cocaine use.
> CLINICIAN 2: You are frustrated with your use.
> CLINICIAN 3: Very fed up…

Simple reflections tend to not alter the direction or theme of conversation. If the dialogue seems stagnant, or the patient keeps repeating himself or herself, it may be time to change from simple to complex reflections.

Complex reflections

This type of reflection adds new words and injects meaning into what was expressed. Complex reflections tend to be more sophisticated and are used as an attempt to infer or add to what the patient might have said, is trying to say, or will say next. This type of reflection allows the clinician to interpret what the patient means or how the patient feels. It is riskier than a simple reflection because it includes material the patient has not clearly said, but it can also be more powerful. Though using complex reflections can be intimidating, a clinician can try to make a reasonable guess based on what is already known about the patient, including clinical context, vulnerabilities, past experiences, and strengths and patterns.

> PATIENT: I had an argument with my daughter today; I started smoking again after three months. I can't believe it.
> CLINICIAN: The argument with your daughter upset you, triggering a relapse, and you ended up disappointing yourself.
> PATIENT: Yes, I feel like a failure again.

In this example, it is not explicitly stated that the patient was first upset and then disappointed; however, the clinician was able to infer these feelings based on the clinical context. The clinician provides a reasonable, educated guess that is not too far away from what the patient was experiencing. Often times, when people are distressed, they have a hard time labeling their emotions. This complex reflection offers two feelings (upset and disappointed) for the patient to explore and permits the clinician to join in and collaboratively help the patient express her thoughts and feelings.

Reflections can intentionally be directed to overstate (emphasize) or understate (downplay) an idea. Miller and Rollnick (2013) explain that if the clinician overstates the intensity of an expressed emotion, the patient would likely minimize and back off from the original statement. On the other hand, if the clinician understates the expressed intensity of an emotion, the patient is likely to continue exploring, providing more information on the subject. It can be useful to overstate or understate when reflecting on an idea, with the goal of prompting the patient to continue talking and exploring. An example of this technique is provided below.

Complex Reflection Overstating the Patient's Idea

> PATIENT: I don't know why my wife keeps nagging me about my drinking.
> CLINICIAN: It is very distressing that she believes that there is something wrong with your drinking, and you don't think there is anything wrong with your drinking.
> PATIENT: I wouldn't say there's nothing wrong with it; I think there is a lot wrong with it. It affects many people and I don't even enjoy it anymore. It's not upsetting; it just bothers me that she brings it up every day.

In the above example, the clinician offers a complex reflection, while also overstating the expressed idea, "you don't think there is anything wrong with your drinking." In turn, the patient is invited to reflect, elaborate more, and provide content that can further enhance and facilitate change.

Complex Reflection Understating the Patient's Idea

PATIENT: Okay, doctor, I am ready! I want to handle this drinking problem. I have had enough.

CLINICIAN: You have some interest to talk about your drinking.

PATIENT: It's not only talking. I want to stop drinking, altogether! It's destroying my marriage.

By contrast, in this example the clinician understates the patient's idea, "You have some interest to talk about your drinking." This allows the patient to verbalize more clearly the intent to stop drinking and the motivation related to the decision, which is to save the marriage. Using statements to overstate or understate an idea allows the patient to elaborate on or clarify any intentions or motivations, which can help with the engagement process.

Summarizing

Summaries are a compilation of statements returned to the patient in multiple reflections or affirmations. Summaries put together thoughts, feelings, and ideas the patient has provided throughout the interview. The clinician should provide a thoughtful and accurate recollection of what was stated, in a way that is helpful for the patient and promotes change. The summation allows the patient to hear his or her own thoughts in a coherent and concise matter. The patient is then invited to approve or correct any information gathered by the clinician, to ensure accuracy and strengthen the relationship. Clinicians should use their intuition and clinical judgment, in the brief moment of deciding when to summarize and what to include in the summary. Ending the summary on a positive note will likely encourage more change. It is often helpful to end with a question that invites the patient to add any other statement to the ones summarized. An example of a clear, concise summary is included in the next section.

EXAMPLES OF USE OF THE CORE SKILLS OF MOTIVATIONAL INTERVIEWING (OARS)

Example 1: Open Question

CLINICIAN: What has happened since we last met?

PATIENT: I've been good, doctor. I have not had a drink since we last met. I did what we talked about and took a different path to work, so I didn't pass by any liquor stores.

Example 2: Affirming

PATIENT: I am so upset with myself. I came home after a long day at work and started drinking. I went without a drink for a month before this, but now I ruined the whole thing. I'm such a loser.

CLINICIAN: It is commendable that you were able to stop drinking for a whole month! Understandably, you're upset about the relapse, but you were able to put together some sober days, which is no small feat.

Example 3: Reflecting

PATIENT: I'm really tired of dealing with this mess of a situation.

CLINICIAN: You've had enough.

PATIENT: I have not had enough. I'm just tired! This is such a mess.

CLINICIAN: A big mess!

PATIENT: Exactly. I feel like my husband and I keep arguing over my drinking and we don't understand each other anymore.

In this interaction, the clinician employs reflections to further understand, and adjusts to the needs of the patient. When the patient is engaged, there is more room for an inaccurate reflection. A well-engaged patient is more likely to allow the clinician to be wrong, without disturbing the flow of the conversation. This enables the clinician to further clarify, allowing for an accurate understanding of the patient's major need or concern, which positively influences the treatment outcome.

Example 4: Summarizing

PATIENT: I felt miserable today.

CLINICIAN: Miserable.

PATIENT: I was thinking about all the skills we discussed in here, but the urges were so great that I couldn't resist. I went to the liquor store and bought a bottle of wine. I didn't drink it though.

CLINICIAN: You didn't drink it.

PATIENT: I did not. I thought about my family, about my little girls.

CLINICIAN: You had a rough day. You tried to put into practice the relapse prevention skills; however, the urge was so great that you ended up going to the liquor store. Your family is very important to you, and you did not want to go home and drink. Instead you came to my office today, to get some support, and stay sober.

In this example, many reflections are included, both simple and complex. The clinician attempts to first understand and then portray the intensity of emotion and thoughts about relapse. The summary ends with two affirmations that invite collaborative problem solving, a key way to remain well engaged with the patient.

Example 5: Using OARS to Enhance Engagement by Clarifying Patient Needs

PATIENT: I don't like coming here because you only focus on getting urine for testing!

CLINICIAN: You would like us to focus on something more important to you.

PATIENT: Everybody here asks how many beers I had last week and whether I used cocaine.

CLINICIAN: Your cocaine and alcohol use is not the only thing to focus on.

PATIENT: I think it is important, but it is not what bothers me the most. I have to think about where I will sleep at night.

CLINICIAN: You are in a very difficult situation. You want help with the most urgent issue for you now, which is your lack of housing.

PATIENT: Exactly. I just want to feel normal, have a house, and get a job. I want to have a family and help people. Do you know what I mean?

CLINICIAN: I do. I understand what you are saying. Thanks for explaining to me the goals you want in life. Once we concentrate on the most acute needs, we may be able to focus on the substance use.

PATIENT: Someone who finally understands me. Exactly correct. That sounds like a good plan.

Example 6: Combining All the Core Skills—OARS—to Promote Engagement

PATIENT: Hi. The court sent me here, I'm not sure I belong here; there's nothing really wrong with me.

CLINICIAN: It's good that you are working with the court recommendations. Can you tell me more about the reason the court sent you here? [*Affirmation and open question*]

PATIENT: They say that my drinking is a problem. I got a DUI. I was just unlucky.

CLINICIAN: Unlucky... [*Simple reflection*]

PATIENT: I'm honest, I drank way more before and they never got me. My wife says I drink too much; I never caused any harm to my family though. I drink a lot with my friends, but I'm able to go to work. Do you know what I mean?

CLINICIAN: Your family and job are important to you. Even when you drink heavily, you manage to keep them out of the problem. [*Affirmation and reflection with understating quality*]

PATIENT: Yes, although this time I got myself into trouble. Don't get me wrong though, I did drink a lot. When I start drinking, before I know it, I lose control and a lot of bad stuff starts to happen.

CLINICIAN: The drinking gets out of control and then it's not fun anymore. It's problematic. [*Complex reflection*]

PATIENT: I guess it is. I don't like to be told what to do though. That's why I hate the court order. I'm my own man. I'm not a kid that you can order around and tell what to do.

CLINICIAN: I'm glad you came, and I commend you for doing so, even when you feel so adamantly against receiving and following orders. [*Affirmation*] What can I do to help? [*Open question*]

PATIENT: You can tell the court that I will be doing whatever I have to do.

CLINICIAN: You would like to do whatever it takes to get the court out of your life. [*Complex reflection*]

PATIENT: If there were a medication to help me cut down on my drinking, I would consider it.

CLINICIAN: You are interested in cutting down on your drinking. [*Simple reflection*]

PATIENT: I mean I can try.

CLINICIAN: That is great that you are willing to try and cut back on your drinking. You drink socially, but it gets to the point where you lose control over your drinking. This gets you into trouble, including conflict with your wife, and now a DUI. You do not appreciate the court's mandate for treatment; however, you are not opposed to participating in treatment to cut down on drinking. [*Summary*]

In this interaction, the patient enters the session upset and apprehensive. He had been mandated to treatment and expects a power difference and hierarchical relationship with the clinician. Through open questions, affirmations, reflections, and a summary, this patient starts to engage in treatment. This interchange reflects OARS and the spirit of MI. The clinician highlights the patient's values and morals, through genuine affirmations. The patient is reminded how important his family and job are, emphasizing the special meaning they have in his life. The patient shows hesitation in the beginning of the conversation; however, as time passes, the patient is able to identify some goals of therapy.

The use of open questions invited exploration, allowing the patient to feel safe and respected and thus provided useful information for the clinician's assessment of the problem. The questions are neither too frequent nor too many, avoiding exhaustion or what sometimes feels like a "checklist." Despite the questions being open, they are not confusing and are focused on the material being discussed. The open questions do not interfere with the natural flow of the conversation. The simple reflections are appropriate and result in more talking. The complex reflections add meaning to the patient's statements and are not too distant from what the patient is saying. Staying on topic and not straying too far from an idea is especially important for a patient in the early stages of engagement.

Overall, this example provides an overview of the fundamental skills of engaging, using OARS—asking open questions, affirming, reflecting, and summarizing—to conduct a mutually respectful interview. Engaging allows a patient to feel valued, heard, and safe to talk about sensitive topics. Within the context of the MI spirit, engaging allows patients to partner with clinicians for the ultimate goal of facilitating change.

KEY POINTS

Goals of Engaging

1. Ensure the patient participates in treatment.

2. Help the patient feel safe to share information.

3. Allow the patient to feel understood, respected, and trusted.

4. Allow the patient to participate in a collaborative way.

Behaviors That Support Engagement

1. Practicing good listening.

2. Providing undivided attention.

3. Comforting with eye contact and genuine facial expression.

Traps to Avoid

1. Excessive questioning.

2. Hierarchical dyad between patient and clinician.

3. Prematurely labeling a patient's problem.

4. Judging and blaming the patient.

5. Excessive chatting.

OARS: Fundamentals of Engaging

Open questions: "How has it been for you since we last met? [*Broad, inviting the patient to elaborate.*]

Affirmations: "It is great that you think about your family." [*Genuine, pointing out the positive, acknowledging strength and values.*]

Reflections: Simple reflection: "Strong cravings" [*Repeating or rephrasing what the patient says*]; Complex reflections: "You are struggling with the cravings" [*Providing an educated guess about the meaning, context, or feeling associated with what the patient said*].

Summaries: "You had increased stress, and it triggered your cravings, which led to you having a couple of drinks. It was good that you returned to the group, to get back on track. Your family is important to you, and you want to continue to work on your sobriety." [*Clear, concise overview, with affirmations and reflections, ending on a positive note.*]

STUDY QUESTIONS

1. Engaging can be considered as

    A. One of the stages of change.
    B. An optional part of motivational interviewing (MI), only necessary for the most difficult patients.
    C. An essential characteristic of the clinician, but does not involve the patient.
    D. One of the four processes in MI, the foundation of every therapeutic relationship.
    E. The end of therapy and is not a prerequisite for the other processes in MI.

2. Which statement is *true* about the core communication skills in MI?

    A. Closed questions should be applied more than open questions.
    B. Open questions promote exploration and facilitate the natural flow of conversation.
    C. A reflection is a core communication skill, but should be used minimally.
    D. Summarizing refers to a compilation of all the flaws and deficits a patient may have.
    E. Affirming is a strategy for depressed patients, to make them feel better.

3. Of the following statements or questions, which one would best promote engagement?

    A. "Your urine toxicology was positive; where did you get the cocaine?"
    B. "I do not think you care about your sobriety. Look at your urine—it's positive."
    C. "I noticed some changes in your urine toxicology this week. Please tell me more about that."
    D. "Your daughter will be disappointed."
    E. "You broke your promise again."

4. Which statement about affirmations is *true*?

    A. They do not have to be genuine.
    B. They are useful only when the patient is considering terminating the treatment.

C. Many should be used in the interview, to make sure the patient likes the clinician.

D. They should be used only after judging the patient for their behaviors.

E. They are genuine and can acknowledge the strengths, values, and inherent worth of patients.

5. Which statement below best describes summarizing?

A. It should not include reflections.

B. It should not include affirmations.

C. It has to be done only when terminating with a patient.

D. It should be provided in a written format.

E. It includes reflections and affirmations and allows the patient to clarify.

REFERENCES

Blatt SJ, Zuroff DC: Empirical evaluation of the assumptions in identifying evidence based treatments in mental health. Clin Psychol Rev 25(4):459–486, 2005 15893862

Bordin ES: The generalizability of the psychoanalytic concept of the working alliance. Psychotherapy: Theory, Research, & Practice 16(3):252–260, 1979

Crits-Christoph P, Hamilton JL, Ring-Kurtz S, et al: Program, counselor, and client variability in the alliance: a multilevel study of the alliance in relation to substance use outcomes. J Subst Abuse Treat 40(4):405–413, 2011

Farrell L, Ingersoll K, Ceperich SD: Enhancing patient adherence: promoting engagement via positive patient-provider relationships in HIV/AIDS care. Med Encount 23(2):69–71, 2009

Fuertes JN, Mislowack A, Bennett J, et al: The physician-patient working alliance. Patient Educ Couns 66(1):29–36, 2007 17188453

Karver MS, Handelsman JB, Fields S, et al: Meta-analysis of therapeutic relationship variables in youth and family therapy: the evidence for different relationship variables in the child and adolescent treatment outcome literature. Clin Psychol Rev 26(1):50–65, 2006 16271815

Martin DJ, Garske JP, Davis MK: Relation of the therapeutic alliance with outcome and other variables: a meta-analytic review. J Consult Clin Psychol 68(3):438–450, 2000 10883561

Miller WR, Rollnick S: Motivational Interviewing: Helping People Change, 3rd Edition. New York, Guilford, 2013

STUDENT REFLECTIONS

Jill Konowich, Ph.D.
Rutgers New Jersey Medical School, MS-IV

Only careful introspection can lead to growth and spur change. This is truly the heart of the engaging process in motivational interviewing (MI). The chapter's opening quote from Carl Rogers calls to this truth as he rephrases his professional goals as "How can I provide a relationship, which this person may use for his own personal growth?" Utilizing MI and fostering a therapeutic clinician-patient relationship is tantamount to providing first-rate medical care. The initial patient encounter involves the divulgence of very private and possibly embarrassing details of the patient's life in order to receive medical care. Engaging the patient provides a comfortable environment for a patient to share personal information and express his or her opinions in a neutral space. I've found that proper engagement can dictate the patient encounter.

I recently had an admitted patient on the surgical floor who was refusing to take his medication, give bloodwork, and sign consent for a life-saving operation. I had yet to meet the patient, but the staff had set the tone that this would be a difficult patient to approach. Instead of falling into the traps that promote disengagement, I came in and sat with the patient and began MI with some open questions. Moreover, I didn't push the team's agenda. This reduced the patient's vulnerability, and, ultimately, our conversation revealed that no one had sat down to explain the operation or the entire situation to the patient. He had felt bombarded by orders and disrespected, which only brewed contempt and distrust for his medical team. The goals of engagement were not met, but by allowing the patient to voice his opinion and participate in his care, he eventually took the necessary steps to do what was best for him and his health.

My experience elucidates the biggest pitfall that leads to failures in MI: a failure to respect autonomy and collaborate with the patient in his or her medical care. I believe physicians always try to follow the Hippocratic oath; however, as time passes, we can get caught up in the process of practicing medicine and forget that at the end of the day, it's the patient's body, and his or her illness, struggles, and choices to make—and it's our job to promote a collaborative environment that ultimately improves the patient's quality of life while preserving autonomy.

Focusing

Grace Kwon, D.O.

> You will never reach your destination if you stop and throw stones at
> every dog that barks.
>
> —*Winston Churchill*

Engaging a patient may be a continual and ongoing process throughout participation in motivational interviewing (MI). But, at some point, you need to
know what you'll do in the session. Sometimes, the direction is very clear. At other
times, the path involving change can be quite challenging and elusive. Using
MI, the clinician facilitates the discussion so the patient chooses a focus based
on his or her motivation to address a specific concern. Many therapeutic techniques have a defined and intentional goal, and in MI the goal is to maintain the
MI spirit while partnering with the patient in change. Focusing is a process that
allows the patient greater specificity for his or her attention. In spending a few
moments to focus the session, you produce a mutually agreed-on area to further
explore the patient's feelings about change. Focusing may not occur as a single step
or in a defined manner, but like the other MI processes, it is an ongoing practice
that allows you to more effectively explore various motivations and behaviors
that a patient identifies as needing change.

This chapter will cover the different sources and styles of focusing in MI.
Steve Jobs said, "Simple can be harder than complex; you have to work hard to
get your thinking clean." Focusing can be deceptively simple, but through the task
of focusing, you can have a more efficient and "clean" path. There may be challenging situations that arise during the focusing process of MI. Clinical examples will be incorporated throughout the chapter to illustrate such challenges.

FOCUSING IN MOTIVATIONAL INTERVIEWING

A patient may have multiple concerns that compete for the focus of his or her attention and ability to make change. For example, let's consider Betty, a 20-year-old single, pregnant woman using drugs, who presents to your office. Once you are confident she is engaged in the process, you can start simply by asking her what she would like to focus on. Keep in mind that the patient may not have a ready list of clear goals. The agenda can include fears, desires, hopes, or other emotional and pragmatic realities. She may have concerns that are related, either directly or indirectly, to her drug use or even her pregnancy, such as

* Concern for the baby's health.
* Fear that the baby may be taken away.
* Shame about drug use during pregnancy.
* Fear of being judged by the medical community or society.
* Anger toward herself.
* Worries about how she will manage financially.

There are many facets at play when you consider the process of focusing, and in keeping with the spirit of MI, allowing for her autonomy, respectfully tolerating uncertainty, and offering information and guidance may be most helpful both in engaging her and in helping her to identify her priorities to focus the conversation.

SOURCES OF FOCUS

There are usually three sources of focus: the patient, the setting, and the clinician. Often the patient is able to provide the direction of focus. An example of this is a patient who comes to you stating he or she wants to quit smoking. The setting, such as a methadone clinic, a weight loss center, or an occupational therapist's office, may provide the focus. And lastly you, the clinician, can provide the source of focusing; however, this should be done while maintaining the spirit of MI. For example, consider a man with hypertension who declines to add a medication for blood pressure control. You are concerned about how his daily alcohol intake is affecting his blood pressure. It may take some artful persuasion, but if you operate in the MI spirit, you can ask if it would be okay to provide information and suggest the direction for focus.

COMMON FOCUSING SCENARIOS

Let's consider the first case. Betty could present to your office with several chief complaints.

Scenario 1: "I'm Pregnant and I'm Going to Stop Using Drugs by Starting Methadone."

Focus and direction are clear.

Sometimes, the patient comes to you with a clear focus and direction. When this happens, you can reflect this to the patient to confirm that the two of you mutually understand the focus of the session. You can proceed to the evoking and planning processes, with reengaging or refocusing, as needed. When the patient states, "I plan to start methadone today," she has a plan and has mobilized change talk consistent with taking steps. If the patient expresses ambivalence, for example, in stating, "I want to start methadone, but I'm afraid I'll feel sick if I stop using heroin," the clinician may choose to engage the patient and reflect the patient's statement. The clinician can show empathy for the patient's worry about what she will experience, while also highlighting the patient's desire to seek treatment—using methadone—in order to maintain the focus on interventions that will help the patient to change the behavior of heroin use during pregnancy. Another option is to offer information about starting methadone and what to expect.

Scenario 2: "I'm Pregnant and I'm Not Sure If I Can Stop Using. I'm Worried About the Baby. I'm Also Scared That the Baby Will Be Taken Away If I Have Drugs in My System When I Deliver."

There are several choices to focus on.

In busy clinical situations, the focusing portion of MI is often done fairly quickly. In this situation, the setting may be influencing the focus of the motivational interview. However, the clinician may find it helpful to reflect the patient's statement, offer an affirmation, and then evoke her preference and motivations. For example, the clinician could say, "There's a lot on your mind. Pregnancy, drug use, and concern over losing the baby are a lot for any one person to manage all at once. It's great that you came in to get started. What would you like to talk about today?" Providing a worksheet such as the one shown in Figure 4–1 can help the clinician facilitate the decision about what to focus on. Remember that focusing in MI is a continuous process in which you and the patient are seeking and maintaining direction. Agenda mapping is one way to facilitate this process (Miller and Rollnick 2013)

Providing a visual aid not only helps the patient organize her concerns and consider what she wants to focus on, but also helps you, the clinician, to understand the breadth of concerns and motivations. You give the patient a template with several empty circles and ask the patient, "What would you like to talk about today?" You can then consider how these agenda items may lead toward goals for the patient. You can use this to then ask the patient to specify which agenda items are most important and pressing. Having a concrete, written form may be of help in prioritizing agenda items for both the patient and you.

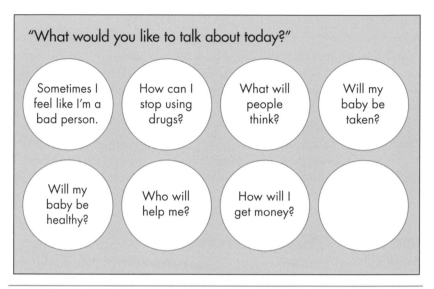

FIGURE 4–1. **Agenda mapping.**

Scenario 3: "I'm Pregnant and I Don't Know If I Want to Keep the Baby. I Don't Know Anything. My Life Is a Mess."

There is no clear focus.

In a case in which the patient has no clear direction, you want to help minimize the confusion. One way you can help the patient is by orienting her. Often, patients present with a history which at times can be difficult to follow. *Orienting* requires you to put the pieces of the patient's story together so that by the end of the session, it is hoped, you will have a patchwork of her whole story. As you'll see in the examples section, this is done by providing a summarized coherent history back to the patient. Having the whole picture will help provide a more comprehensive understanding of the patient's current circumstances and how she might want to proceed.

In a scenario where the patient has no clear focus, the clinician can facilitate the conversation to assist the patient in identifying several loci of possible focus as in scenario 2. Then, the clinician can use agenda mapping or other techniques as appropriate to assist in determining the focus.

One such technique that may be of help is *zooming in*, a term used by Miller and Rollnick (2013). Imagine using an Internet map to find the place you plan to travel to. Just like pushing the (+) button to zoom in and the (-) button to zoom out, you can zoom in and out of the big picture of the patient's situation to focus in or out. Often zooming in and focusing on a starting point helps you and the patient navigate through the map to a destination.

ADDITIONAL METHODS TO CONSIDER

Elicit-Provide-Elicit

This is a strategy that can be employed when the clinician would like to provide some information in a respectful and collaborative way to the patient. The clinician first elicits knowledge that the patient has. The second step is to provide information to the patient in a clear and MI-consistent manner. Finally, the clinician elicits the patient's reaction to the presented information to see if he or she understands the content and has processed it.

Changing Direction

Another concept to consider in any of the scenarios above is termed *changing direction*. Periodically, a patient presents with a goal in mind, and on the basis of the clinician's clinical expertise, the clinician decides to set a goal that diverges quite a bit from the goal set forth by the patient. Approaching this difference in goals, especially if the clinician's goal introduces a difficult subject, can be quite challenging. The clinician should reiterate the patient's goals, respect the patient's autonomy, and transparently ask for permission to introduce a new goal, while providing the rationale for doing so.

SPECIAL CONSIDERATIONS

Ethics

Usually, there is a power differential that exists in the professional relationship between the patient and the clinician. It is important to operate within the broad medical ethical principles of nonmaleficence, beneficence, autonomy, and justice (Beauchamp and Childress 2001). When using MI, the clinician should be mindful of situations in which use of MI would not be consistent with these principles. For example,

> Dr. Lee owns "Rehab Center" and he uses MI to resolve ambivalence about which rehabilitation center the patient will go to for his or her cocaine use disorder after the patient has already decided to enter treatment.

Decision to Self-Disclose

It is not an uncommon phenomenon for a patient to be curious about the clinician. Ultimately, the clinician has to make a decision about whether to share personal information. If the clinician chooses to disclose personal information, the clinician also has to decide how much information about his or her private lives to divulge. In MI, the clinician should first and foremost operate under the ethical principles outlined earlier in the subsection "Ethics." The clinician should consider whether the disclosure will be beneficial to the patient-clinician relationship and whether it will promote collaboration and trust.

EXAMPLES OF USE OF FOCUSING IN MOTIVATIONAL INTERVIEWING

The following three narratives correspond to examples of the focusing scenarios for Betty described earlier in this chapter. An additional scenario illustrating changing direction is provided.

Scenario 1: Focus and Direction Are Clear

CLINICIAN: What brings you in to our clinic today?

PATIENT: I am pregnant, using heroin, and I want to stop.

CLINICIAN: You would like to stop using heroin now that you are pregnant. What options have you considered?

PATIENT: I heard from my friends methadone works so I don't get sick. I want my baby to be healthy, and I want to be a good mom. I'm ready to stop.

CLINICIAN: You'd like your baby to be healthy and you are taking steps to be a good mom, starting with methadone. You've heard about methadone helping to prevent withdrawal from a friend. It's great that you are seeking treatment. Can I share with you information about methadone, and all your other non-medication and medication options, including buprenorphine?

PATIENT: That sounds great! Come to think of it, I heard one of my friends talk about buprenorphine, and she did really well on it. I read something about it on the Internet, and I'd love to find out more information about it.

CLINICIAN: Wonderful. The focus of this visit will be to provide you with information about treatment options for opioid use disorder during pregnancy. We'll also explore what best fits your situation given your reasons for taking this step, and then come up with a plan about where to go from here.

Scenario 2: There Are Several Choices to Focus On

CLINICIAN: You were referred to me for possible treatment with methadone, and you have a lot of other things on your mind. You talked about how you wanted to keep the baby, and you want to minimize harm to the baby. You also mentioned your concern that your baby could be removed from your care if you continue using drugs. Where should we start?

PATIENT: Yes, I'm very worried about these things. I have a lot on my mind. I really want the baby to be safe.

CLINICIAN: You would like to focus on ways to keep the baby well and safe.

PATIENT: Yes, and I understand that these issues are related. I know I need to get the right treatment to stop using. Being sober will help me take care of myself and the baby, and stay focused on what's important. I have heard about treatment with methadone and buprenorphine, but I also need to know how they will affect my baby.

CLINICIAN: You want the right treatment, and we've spoken about the role of medications. At the same time, it's important to understand how medications can affect the baby. What do you already know?

Scenario 3: There Is No Clear Focus

CLINICIAN: There are a lot of things going on in your life right now. Just to make sure I understand, let me summarize what you have told me thus far. You just found out you are pregnant during your visit to the emergency room. This is your first pregnancy, and you don't know what to do. You were in the emergency room because your boyfriend assaulted you, but it is important for you to stay with him because he is the father of your baby. You're worried because you don't have any financial support now. You feel that heroin use helps you to escape the stressors of your life.

PATIENT: It's the only thing working for me in my life right now.

CLINICIAN: Heroin has been the only reliable thing in your life recently.

PATIENT: Well, I feel better after I use, but it may not be reliable. I did end up in the emergency room a few weeks ago because I overdosed. I worry that is going to affect my baby.

CLINICIAN: You're concerned about how heroin use and an overdose affect the baby.

PATIENT: Of course I am. This is my first pregnancy, and as much as I don't want to think about it, I smile at the thought of being a good mother.

CLINICIAN: Even though your life is chaotic right now, thinking about the possibility of being a good mother brings you joy.

PATIENT: Yes, I want to be a good mother. But, it's all too much to think about; I have too much going on.

CLINICIAN: There's a lot to balance at once. It's hard to sort out where to start, but becoming a mother and starting a new life brings opportunity for positive change in your life.

PATIENT: Yes, I want this baby, and I would like to turn my life around.

Through orienting the patient, the clinician brings the focus to the beginning of scenario 2, where he or she can implement structuring, consider options, and use zooming in.

Scenario 4: Changing Direction

PATIENT: I want to lose weight, Doc. Summer is coming up, and I want to look good on the beach.

CLINICIAN: You're ready to lose some weight.

PATIENT: I've been doing everything you told me to last time, including exercising 30 minutes every day with some cardio and some weightlifting.

CLINICIAN: It's great you've followed the plan you made for yourself during our last appointment. How did the meeting with the dietician go earlier in the week?

PATIENT: It went well. Now I understand what foods I should avoid later in the day.

CLINICIAN: You made a lot of progress doing exercise and understanding how your eating patterns can affect your ability to lose weight. You came here because you wanted to lose weight. You've made plans about diet and certain exercise regimens you have incorporated into your daily schedule. We can continue to talk about these options, and another option is to talk about how your alcohol intake may be contributing to your overall health and weight. Would that be okay with you?

EXAMPLES OF APPROACHES INCONSISTENT AND CONSISTENT WITH MOTIVATIONAL INTERVIEWING

A 65-year-old male with cirrhosis presents to the emergency room with a blood alcohol level of 0.310 g/dL. The following day, you are consulted for management of alcohol use disorder.

MI–Inconsistent Approaches

PATIENT: I don't know what happened yesterday, but my stomach hurts. When can I leave?

CLINICIAN: The primary team consulted me on your alcohol use disorder. How much do you drink daily?

PATIENT: Uhh…I don't drink every day. Maybe I drink every other day.

CLINICIAN: How much? What kind of alcohol do you like to drink?

PATIENT: Maybe I take about 5 shots of whiskey every other day.

CLINICIAN: When did you start drinking?

PATIENT: I think I was about 13 years old.

CLINICIAN: Do you use any other substances?

PATIENT: No.

CLINICIAN: Do you smoke?

PATIENT: Yes.

CLINICIAN: How much and how long?

PATIENT: About a pack since I was about 13 years old.

CLINICIAN: What are the consequences of your drinking? Do you have any legal issues?

PATIENT: I think my liver's given out on me. I had two DUIs in the past four years.

CLINICIAN: Do you think your drinking is a problem?

PATIENT: No. Well maybe a little, but it's what everyone in my family does.

Besides, it's not like I drink every single day and it's not like I've had seizures.

CLINICIAN: Would you want medications to help you stop drinking?

PATIENT: I don't really want to stop drinking.

MI-Consistent Approaches (Using Elicit-Provide-Elicit)

PATIENT: I don't know what happened yesterday, but my stomach hurts. When can I leave?

CLINICIAN: You are in a lot of pain and are somewhat perplexed about the events that led to your hospital admission.

PATIENT: Yeah, I was at a friend's house and we were having some whiskey and playing cards. I must have passed out and somehow ended up here.

CLINICIAN: Would it be okay with you if I chronicle the events that led to your admission?

PATIENT: Sure, because I have no idea.

CLINICIAN: From the information that the primary team told me, you lost consciousness and were vomiting blood. Your friend then called 911.

PATIENT: Oh. Vomiting blood? My stomach has been hurting. Where was the blood from?

CLINICIAN: I'll answer that question for you, but I just want to make sure that you've understood what I've told you thus far. Can you tell me what happened?"

PATIENT: I passed out, vomited blood, and came to the emergency room.

CLINICIAN: Okay, I wanted to confirm you understood me. Now back to your question. The blood is likely from ruptured varices in your esophagus.

PATIENT: What are varices? Why did they rupture?

CLINICIAN: From the information in your medical history and laboratory results, you have cirrhosis of the liver. The scarring from cirrhosis prevents the blood from going through the liver, and this can cause a "backup" in the veins around the esophagus. They become fragile and can rupture with pressure such as during vomiting. You came in to the emergency room with a blood alcohol level of 0.310 g/dL. Consistent alcohol use is a common cause for the cirrhosis of the liver. Tell me your thoughts.

PATIENT: Alcohol…Yeah…I guess I've been on a bender for the past couple of months. I've been drinking almost every day. I didn't know alcohol could make you throw up blood. I like drinking to forget my problems and feel relaxed, but I never thought I'd end up here for something like this.

CLINICIAN: It's scary to think that something that started as a way to escape problems and feel relaxed may now be causing you to have serious health problems and end up in the ER.

PATIENT: Yeah, and my dad, well, he died from his liver giving out on him. And my family doc has been on my case about my liver. I guess I have the same thing my dad had.

CLINICIAN: I'm sorry to hear about your father. From what you are saying, his drinking contributed to his death, and you don't want the same thing to happen to you since you may have the same problem.

PATIENT: It killed him.... It could kill me. Who are you again?

CLINICIAN: I'm Dr. Seo and I was called by the primary team because they are concerned about your health and your use of alcohol. It sounds like you have given your alcohol use some thought already.

PATIENT: Do you think it's killing me, doc? I've tried to stop on my own a couple of times but I just couldn't.

CLINICIAN: Your alcohol use is definitely contributing to your current health problems, and we can think of ways to help you stop. There are even medications that can help. Would you be interested in hearing about them?

KEY POINTS

- There are three sources of focus: the patient, the setting, and the clinician. There are three common focusing scenarios:

  1. Focus and direction are clear.

  2. There are several choices to focus on (the focus is not clear).

  3. There is no clear focus (the direction is unclear).

- Start with orienting and once a few options come into view, you can use the following strategies to get the focus to become clearer:

  - Agenda mapping

  - Zooming in

  - Elicit-provide-elicit

  - Changing direction

- Keep in mind the four aspects of the spirit of MI when focusing: partnership, acceptance, compassion, and evocation.

STUDY QUESTIONS

1. Which strategy is used when the patient has a goal that is far from the goal the clinician would like to discuss?

    A. Elicit-provide-elicit.
    B. Changing direction.
    C. Agenda mapping.
    D. Zooming in.
    E. Orienting.

2. A 30-year-old women presents to your office stating her life is completely in shambles. Which of the following is a technique to use in focusing during motivational interviewing (MI)?

   A. Zooming in.
   B. Imagining.
   C. Helping.
   D. Zoning out.
   E. Picturing.

3. Which of the following questions can begin the process of agenda mapping?

   A. What is your psychiatric history?
   B. What is the chronological timeline for your presenting problem?
   C. Can you draw a few circles and write what you would like to discuss today?
   D. Where did we end the session last week?
   E. What would you like to talk about today?

4. Which of the following scenarios would be considered unethical use of motivational interviewing (MI)?

   A. The patient has no focus and tells you a story that is very difficult to follow.
   B. The patient does not want to change.
   C. You are offered money in exchange for your clinical expertise.
   D. A CEO asks you to use MI to help bring patients to an intensive outpatient program in exchange for a medical directorship.
   E. A doctor consults you to talk to a diabetic patient about his poorly controlled blood glucose.

5. How does agenda mapping help the clinician using MI?

   A. Makes your life easier.
   B. Allows you to pick something quickly.
   C. Helps the clinician map out the session.
   D. Helps the clinician understand the breadth of possible agendas on which the patient may want to focus the conversation.
   E. Gives insight into the psyche of the patient.

REFERENCES

Beauchamp TL, Childress JF: Principles of Biomedical Ethics, 5th Edition. New York, Oxford University Press, 2001

Miller WR, Rollnick S: Motivational Interviewing: Helping People Change, 3rd Edition. New York, Guilford, 2013

STUDENT REFLECTIONS

Eli Neustadter
Yale School of Medicine, MS2

As a current medical student and aspiring psychiatrist, I found this chapter helpful in highlighting the conceptual and ethical principles underlying motivational interviewing (MI) and providing practical guidance for focusing during the clinical encounter. Underlying MI is the foundational principle of autonomy, and the current discussion on "focusing" demonstrated to me how it can be an effective tool for partnering with the patient and orienting the clinician to what is of greatest importance to the patient. This chapter also taught me how focusing can be an effective tool for "zooming in" on actionable problems when a patient may be facing many biopsychosocial concerns that cannot all be addressed in a single encounter.

In psychiatry, as in other medical contexts, patients may have varying degrees of insight into their condition as well as different degrees of specification for how they want to achieve their goals. The patient-clinician scenarios provided in the chapter will be a great resource to me as I enter into wards and begin to devise action plans with patients. Each scenario in the chapter presents a case in which the patient has more or less directedness in how he or she wants to address his or her concerns and demonstrates how a variety of MI techniques (e.g. agenda mapping, orienting, elicit-provide-elicit) can be employed to help the patient come to a better understanding of his or her condition. Moreover, focusing can help the clinician partner with his or her patient to change the patient's perception of what appears to be an overwhelming circumstance (in the current chapter, a pregnant woman using heroin with concerns about her fetus's health) into a set of prioritized and manageable goals (e.g., explore pregnancy-safe treatment options for heroin dependency).

▶Chapter

5

Evoking

Mandrill Taylor, M.D., M.P.H.

> We have ways to make men talk.
> —*Mohammed Khan in* The Lives of a Bengal Lancer *(1935)*

> No matter what anybody tells you, words and ideas can change the world.
> —*John Keating in* Dead Poets Society *(1989)*

Evoking motivation by enhancing both the importance of change and one's confidence in the ability to change is a hallmark of motivational interviewing (MI). In order to utilize this general MI process of evoking change in clinical practice, one must be able to recognize change talk and respond to it accordingly.

This chapter will expand on the various ways one can begin to *recognize* the various types of ambivalence, change talk, sustain talk, and discord, which can all occur at any given point within a conversation. Once these concepts have been recognized, one must also learn how best to *respond* in a manner that reinforces change toward action rather than providing instruction, which could elicit either counterarguments or interpersonal discord. Lastly, this chapter will address ways to *evoke* motivation and/or confidence if no form of change talk has occurred through use of structured recognition and response techniques.

RECOGNIZE

Ambivalence

Quite often, delayed decisions are associated with a certain degree of ambivalence, which makes taking action difficult. *Ambivalence* is contemplation of conflicting motivations for and against change. Effectively promoting positive change requires recognition of ambivalence, which comes in many forms (Figure 5–1).

Win-Win ☺☺	Also known as "champagne problems," win-win decisions will result in a positive outcome with either choice. The stress comes with making the most beneficial decision.
Lose-Lose ☹☹	Also known as "between a rock and a hard place," lose-lose decisions lead to negative outcomes with either choice. The stress results from attempting to minimize discomfort.
Win & Lose ☺ ☹	Also known as "push-pull," sometimes the decision is between maintaining the status quo or making a change, which may cause stress once benefits of the status quo or consequences of that change are further realized.
Win & Lose ☺☺ ☹☹	Exploring more than one complex option can be especially stressful as one may find oneself in constant flux, being pushed to one option due to consequences of the other or being pulled back to that option due to its potential benefits.

FIGURE 5–1. **Types of ambivalence.**

Regardless of its nature, ambivalence can affect one's motivation. In moving toward action, disadvantages of that action become more apparent, and this can prevent change from occurring. Therefore, MI places the focus back on the advantages through use of change talk. However, one must be able to recognize change talk in others in order to evoke their own personal motivation.

Change Talk

Change talk represents shared thoughts on arguments toward action. The concept is simple: a good predictor of future action is arguing on its behalf—the more a person argues on behalf of an action, the more likely he or she is to go through with it. Miller and Rollnick (2013) describe change talk as a two-sided hill, which consists of preparation on the uphill side and mobilization on the downhill side. More specifically, preparatory change talk focuses on the advantages of change, whereas mobilizing change talk focuses on resolution of ambivalence through commitment and subsequent preparation (the latter of which will be discussed in more detail in Chapter 6, "Planning").

Several different subtypes of change talk, as categorized by motivational psycholinguist Paul Amrhein (1992), are discussed in the following subsections. In understanding the varying degrees of commitment language, one will be in a much better position to assess willingness and promote readiness toward change.

Preparatory Change Talk

Desire

Communicating desire for change is one of the ways that an individual provides a window of opportunity to enhance his or her own motivation. Desire statements usually begin with "I *wish*," "I *want*," or "I'd *like*." They communicate preferences—for example, "I *want* to stop smoking." By expressing desire for change, the individual has opened a door toward exploring his or her ambivalence with stopping smoking. It is through this means that recognizing change talk can lead to commitment for action for someone who remains on the fence.

Ability

Communicating ability for change is yet another way that change talk toward preparation can occur. Ability statements usually begin with "I *can*" or "I *could*." Such statements communicate capacity—for example, "I *could* try walking more." In acknowledging an ability to walk more, the individual is saying that doing so is a possibility. If you can acknowledge walking more is possible, you can subsequently commit to making that happen.

Reasons

Stating reasons for change allows for specific arguments encouraging action to occur. Sometimes the reasons are implied in desire statements—for example, "I would like to live longer." Although "I would like" is a desire statement, "to live longer" is a reason for change. Unlike our first example desire statement, "I want to stop smoking," in which an action of change was stated, living longer is not explicitly an action. Living longer is the result of behavioral change. However, at other times, reasons for behavioral change are explicitly stated: "Eating less meat would lower my cholesterol." Understanding these various forms of preparatory talk can better assist you in identifying opportunities for assisting someone in health-promoting behavioral change.

Need

Utilizing imperative language communicates a sense of obligation in making commitments toward change. These statements usually begin with "I need" or "I've got to." They communicate a sense of urgency—for example, "I need to stop drinking." There is an undertone of moral responsibility and obligation that accompanies the use of need statements, which can be a powerful motivation for change, if properly identified.

Mobilizing Change Talk

Commitment

Mobilizing change talk begins with commitment. These statements usually begin with "I will," "I guarantee," or "I vow." They communicate dedication—for example, "I'm going to the gym." Compared with preparatory change talk, this statement conveys a higher likelihood of action. Commitment talk is the language of verbal contract, signifying an expectation of intention.

Activation

Activation language can be the precursor to commitment language, which requires distinctly different responses. Therefore, distinguishing its difference from commitment talk becomes important in properly enhancing motivation. These statements usually begin with "I'm willing" or "I'm ready." They communicate a sense of commitment without actually fully committing—for example, "It's time to put my health first." Activation language can be an important conduit in mobilizing change. However, mistaking activation for commitment can stall the process. If you begin taking steps toward preparation without the person having expressed commitment language, he or she is less likely to actually go through with the plan discussed. Therefore, when activation language is recognized, it is important to use open questions to elicit specifics, which we'll discuss in more detail in the section "Respond" later in this chapter. Through elaboration, activation language can evolve into commitment talk, which should remain a goal.

Taking steps

Recognizing someone's efforts in preparing for change is also important—for example, "I didn't purchase drugs last week." Identifying steps made toward change creates an opportunity to strengthen motivation through use of affirmation, which will also be discussed in the section "Respond" later in this chapter.

Sustain Talk

In the third edition of their book on motivational interviewing, Miller and Rollnick (2013) discard the concept of resistance and deconstruct it into two overlapping, yet distinct phenomena: sustain talk and discord. *Sustain talk* constitutes arguing to preserve the status quo, and while it does occur in an interpersonal context, it signifies ambivalence, rather than a strain in the therapeutic alliance. *Discord*, on the other hand, may occur in the context of ambivalence, but primarily points to an interpersonal problem, rather than a reluctance to entertain change.

Sustain talk represents shared arguments against action. It is a natural occurrence that can result in response to exploring reasons for behavioral change. However, the more sustain talk is explored, the more likely sustained behavior will result. Therefore, recognizing sustain talk becomes just as important as recognizing change talk in being able to provide the appropriate response.

"I just enjoy eating out." [*Desire*]
"I won't be able to quit with all this stress going on right now." [*Ability*]
"Getting high calms my nerves." [*Reasons*]
"I need to drink alcohol to sleep at night." [*Need*]
"I'm going to the casino this weekend." [*Commitment*]
"I'm not ready to stop smoking yet." [*Activation*]
"I did not renew my gym membership." [*Taking steps*]

You may have noticed that each example of sustain talk is associated with a different subtype of change talk. Essentially, sustain talk is the opposite of change talk.

Discord

Ambivalence results from intrapsychic conflict that can sometimes co-occur with and aggravate interpersonal tension. In other words, people become upset if they feel they are being forced or manipulated, which is not the goal of MI. MI should be used to help enhance the motivation of others, not to control them. Rifts within the therapeutic alliance should be recognized and rectified at face value, rather than explained away as patient resistance.

Let's review some signals of discord to better identify potential barriers in enhancing motivational change.

Defensiveness

Defensiveness comes in many forms and may occur in the course of performing MI at some point or another. Therefore, it is important for us to identify its many manifestations—for example, "I'm only smoking half a pack."

Minimizing is a common response and allows the patient to reframe his or her unhealthy behavior in a way that reduces the urgency for change. If the problem is not serious, then there is less need to address it—for example, "I drink daily because I have anxiety issues."

Another form of defensiveness is rationalization. Justifying reasons for unhealthy behavior can also prevent change from occurring. Many times, this justification will come in a seemingly logical manner. Although logic may explain behavior, it may not always provide validation for it—for example, "Living with that woman causes me to get high."

Blaming is also a common way to express defensiveness. Placing the responsibility for one's action on another can facilitate helplessness in creating a perception that making change is also the responsibility of another.

Squaring Off

Some may perceive MI as being confrontational, which may trigger a response of opposition. This reaction is often accompanied with "you" statements to signify the division in alliance—for example, "You don't know my life." Identifying the power struggle allows one to bypass it by not responding with arguing, which can further split the relationship.

Interrupting

Interrupting can come in the form of someone actually interrupting you or through language that highlights antipathy—for example, "I'm not ready to quit smoking." Recognizing this form of discord is important, as it is an indication someone is feeling influenced.

Disengagement

Like interrupting, disengagement can also come in multiple forms; both verbal and nonverbal. Someone can change the topic or just simply look away while you are speaking—for example, "It's getting late." Disengagement can be quite simple. It can also feel quite dismissive. However, one must remain strategic in responding to discord. We will discuss this topic further in the following section ("Respond").

RESPOND

After gaining the ability to identify ambivalence, change talk, sustain talk, and discord, one must learn how to respond in a manner that helps the therapeutic alliance and reinforces the person's desire for change. Motivation occurs in an interpersonal context and can be enhanced or weakened on the basis of the responses of others. Therefore, this section provides a discussion of how to facilitate change talk and how to help minimize sustain talk. It also addresses the issue of interpersonal discord, which may occur during the response process.

Change Talk

Now that you are comfortable identifying the various forms of change talk, let's discuss how you might respond to such language, using the framework of OARS (open questions, affirmations, reflections, summaries).

Asking Open Questions

When the clinician asks open questions, the patient is more likely to provide a more in-depth response; the more in-depth the response, the greater the opportunity for change. Two specific types of open question effective in progressing MI are *elaboration* and *providing examples*.

PATIENT: I don't make the best decisions when I drink.
CLINICIAN: How do these decisions affect you?

PATIENT: I don't make the best decisions when I drink.
CLINICIAN: Tell me an example of when that last happened.

When you ask for more details or examples, the response likely will lead to more change talk.

Affirming

Affirming someone's change talk provides positive reinforcement and increases its likelihood of evolving into action.

PATIENT: I need to stop gambling.
CLINICIAN: I'm glad you're addressing this.

Affirmations are simple responses, which can have a profound effect in placing focus on areas of change.

Reflecting

Reflective statements are one of the most powerful tools in MI and can range from simple to complex.

PATIENT: I need to eat start eating healthy.
CLINICIAN: Your health is important to you.

The take-home message is when you hear change talk, reflect it, and you are then likely to hear more of it.

A simple reflection can be as simple as repeating or rephrasing what was said to place emphasis on certain words. A complex reflection may involve interpretation, which can potentially have a more meaningful impact. Reflective statements will be discussed in more detail in a later subsection ("Reflective Responses to Sustain Talk").

Summarizing

Providing reflective summaries allows us to revisit and examine the change talk expressed.

CLINICIAN: Alcohol has caused you a lot of stress. You'd like to quit and have listed several reasons why you should. You've also already made steps toward cutting down and listed your family as a strong motivation to change.

It is helpful to reflect both thoughts and emotions to make a more salient connection with an individual.

Sustain Talk

Although the use of reflective statements in encouraging change talk has already been discussed, we now focus on how to use such statements as well as other strategies to respond to sustain talk. Let's look at some examples of those responses below.

Reflective Responses to Sustain Talk

Basic reflections

Repeating or rephrasing someone else's sustain talk can actually facilitate change talk.

> PATIENT: I don't have difficulties with alcohol.
> CLINICIAN: Alcohol hasn't caused you any difficulties.
> PATIENT: Well, my wife thinks it's an issue.

Although the patient originally denies alcohol use is a problem, he subsequently acknowledges possible marital discord after hearing his own words rephrased by someone else. At times, it is easier to identify the discrepancy in our own thoughts if we hear them in someone else's voice.

Amplified reflections

Increasing the magnitude of someone else's sustain talk can also elicit them to engage in change talk.

> PATIENT: I don't have a drinking problem.
> CLINICIAN: Alcohol has never caused you any problems in life.
> PATIENT: Well, "never" is a strong word. It has caused me some problems.

Through use of amplified language, the patient is compelled to correct the clinician, which leads the patient to vocalizing reasons for change. Now, the clinician can respond and elicit further change talk.

Double-sided reflections

Use of this technique highlights discrepancy by combining a reflective statement of sustain talk with previously stated change talk.

> PATIENT: Just because I drink daily, that doesn't mean I have a problem.
> CLINICIAN: You enjoy drinking beer every day, and at the same time, you want
>   to lose weight.

Note that the doctor first restates the patient's sustain talk and then restates the patient's previously mentioned change talk. This technique provides improved saliency in remembering desire for change. The doctor also utilizes "and" rather than "yet" or "but," which may have increased the likelihood of interpersonal discord.

Strategic Responses To Sustain Talk

Emphasizing autonomy

Simply acknowledging someone's autonomy can have a profound effect on reducing sustain talk.

> PATIENT: I'm just not ready to stop smoking.
> CLINICIAN: And that's your choice. Only you can choose to quit smoking.

Emphasizing autonomy minimizes fear of coercion, which can occur if sustain talk is confronted too aggressively.

Reframing

Changing one's perspective on a situation can also facilitate behavioral change.

> PATIENT: I tried to quit smoking before, but then I relapsed after a year.
> CLINICIAN: You stopped smoking for a year; that's impressive.

Reframing the patient's self-doubt allows her to see the previously unseen potential for change. Note that the doctor did not judge the patient's perception; just merely provided an alternative one.

Agreeing with a twist

Providing a reflective statement prior to reframing the sustain talk is another way to facilitate change talk.

> PATIENT: Unemployment has been so stressful. It's just not a good time to quit smoking.
> CLINICIAN: Smoking can help with stress. Purchasing cigarettes with limited finances can definitely cause stress.

Tread lightly with this technique. Your reframed statement should be said in passing and without inflection. It can be very effective, but there is a risk of interpersonal discord if interpreted as adversarial.

Running head start

Asking someone to list their reasons for sustaining behavior can help lead them into a discussion focused on the associated consequences and benefits of change.

> PATIENT: I only smoke cigarettes when I drink.
> CLINICIAN: Quitting is not a priority for you.
> PATIENT: I just like having a good time when I go out.

> CLINICIAN: You're just trying to have fun and only smoke when you go out drinking.
> PATIENT: Yeah.
> CLINICIAN: What may be some disadvantages?
> PATIENT: Well, cigarettes aren't cheap and I usually wake up with a sore throat the next day.

This technique can be effective if change talk is scarce. Engaging in sustain talk can promote objectivity in evaluating need for change.

Now that we have discussed how one responds to sustain talk, let's move on to how one recognizes and responds to interpersonal discord.

Discord

Responding to discord is of vital importance because it can sever alliance, which is the conduit to change. Let us review the varied styles of response one can give in the face of discord.

Reflecting

Much as in responding to sustain talk, reflective statements remain an excellent strategy in addressing verbal barriers to change, like interpersonal discord. For example, the patient says, "I don't think you have enough experience to help me." This is a classic squaring off statement that signals the presence of interpersonal discord. As stated in the subsection on sustain talk, reflective responses can come in several forms: basic, amplified, and double-sided.

- *Basic:* "You don't feel I have the experience to help you."
- *Amplified:* "You feel that I can't help you in any way."
- *Double-sided:* "You came here for help, and you're concerned whether I can help you."

Each one of these types of reflective statements communicates something different and has its place in mending the therapeutic alliance.

Using Strategic Responses

Responses used to respond to sustain talk can also be used in addressing interpersonal discord. As stated before, emphasizing autonomy minimizes fear of coercion, which could be fueling the disagreement. Reframing helps to change one's perspective, and agreeing with a twist provides a unique opportunity to both reflect and reframe.

Apologizing

Another response technique is apologizing. Sometimes just acknowledging one's role in the discord can greatly reduce its impact on the relationship. One can say, "I'm sorry. I misunderstood." It's a simple approach that communicates well-meaning intentions.

Affirming

Although this technique was originally discussed as a means of encouraging change talk, it may also be used as a means of responding to discord. Affirmations can reduce the patient's defensiveness as they communicate collaborative intentions—for example, "You've worked hard to open up about some difficult things in your past."

Redirecting

Redirecting someone can be very effective and also communicates collaborative intention. Sometimes individuals may misinterpret your intentions and would benefit from a shift in conversation, as further inaccurate conclusions may develop from the misinterpretation. For example, you could say, "I'm not interested in assigning blame. My goal is to help you." Although you could directly refute someone's interpretation of you and your intentions, it may also result in further discord. Utilizing softer language may better facilitate emotional de-escalation, which can derail the therapeutic relationship.

EVOKE

Although recognizing and responding to change talk is the cornerstone of MI, what does one do if change talk appears not to be present? There are several reasons why this could be the case. A person could be silently contemplating change. Whether because of introversion or lack of sufficient alliance, many individuals may not initially engage in change talk even if ambivalence is present. Therefore, evoking a person's own motivations for such change is an important step in being able to utilize the techniques discussed in the previous section.

Using Evocation Questions

If change talk is not present, one should consider evoking such talk through the use of open questions. As previously stated (see "Asking Open Questions" in the subsection "Change Talk"), open questions are likely to provide a more in-depth response; the more in-depth the response, the greater the opportunity for change.

In order to generate preparatory change talk, ask questions using the same language. If you want to evoke someone's *desire* for change, ask about his or her desire for change. If you want to evoke someone's *reasons* for change, ask about his or her reasons for change.

Evoking Importance of Making a Behavioral Change

Let's expand on evoking someone's *need* for change. Asking someone about the importance of change can be a very powerful motivator. However, one should do so in a manner that generates a response that encourages self-talk toward change.

Butler et al. (1999) found that asking someone to rate the importance of making behavioral change was effective in evoking preparatory change talk (Figure 5–2).

> On a scale from 0 to 10, 0 being "not at all important" and 10 being "extremely important," how important is it for you to exercise more?

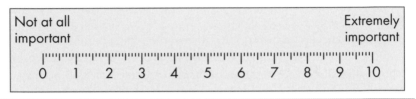

FIGURE 5–2.   Importance ruler.

Resist the urge to ask patients why they did not rate the need for change higher. It may seem natural to convince someone that healthy behavioral change should be important. However, if someone is ambivalent, there may be a tendency for him or her to find reasons to argue against your suggestions, which reinforces sustain talk. In order to avoid that pitfall, simply ask the patient why he or she did not rate the need for change lower. "You rated your need for change as a 2; why didn't you rate it as a 1?" The patient's response will more than likely come in the form of change talk. You now have a front-row seat to someone talking himself or herself into change. If someone states 0, then ambivalence does not currently exist. Therefore, you need to develop discrepancy between the perception and reality of the situation. "What would it take for it to go from 0 to 2?" Although we will discuss evoking motivation in more detail later in the chapter (see subsection "Finding Motivation"), this is an effective follow-up to better ensure the likelihood of change. This statement can be used anytime the patient does not rate the need for change at 10.

Querying Extremes

Exploring the worst consequences of sustained behaviors and the best outcomes of behavioral change can also evoke change talk. This approach is another example of someone talking himself or herself into change rather than being talked into it by someone else.

Looking Back/Looking Forward

Looking back and recalling life before unhealthy decisions were made can facilitate change talk by placing focus on the divergence between the present and the possible.

What were some of the reasons you chose to exercise in the past?

What was life like before you started drinking daily?

If healthy behavior was possible in the past, then it is also possible in the present. If someone's responses highlight even worse difficulties than in the present, then focus on the progress that has been made since that time.

Looking forward and envisioning a brighter future can also help bring about change talk. One could also look forward and envision a dire future if unhealthy behavior is sustained. For example, you could ask, "If you stopped smoking, how would your life be different?" This latter technique of looking forward is similar to querying extremes but differs in that realistic analysis is being requested rather than merely a best-case scenario.

Evoking and Enhancing Confidence

These evoking techniques are effective under the assumption that both confidence and some degree of motivation are present. However, what if that were not the case? What if someone overcame some ambivalence yet had little confidence in actually making a change? These are very real scenarios that occur in clinical practice. Even if someone can see the importance of change, change is less likely to occur without confidence in being able to execute the action. The following techniques can facilitate evocation and enhancement of confidence when it is absent.

Asking Open Questions: Confidence Talk

As stated earlier in the subsection "Change Talk" (see section "Respond"), asking open questions allows the respondent to provide more in-depth responses, which leads to greater opportunity to discover. For example, you could ask, "What problems would you anticipate, and how would you overcome them?" Confidence can be enhanced through mental preparation. Also, responding to answers with reflective statements can help to reinforce emerging confidence.

Determining Level of Confidence in Ability to Change: Confidence Ruler

Much like asking the importance of change, inquiring about someone's confidence in being able to make that change can also be a powerful motivator. Such inquiries create an environment where subsequent responses can lead someone toward change talk.

The confidence ruler (Figure 5–3) can be used to determine a patient's level of confidence in being able to change, much as the importance ruler can be used to rate the importance of change.

On a scale from 0 to 10, 0 being "not at all confident" and 10 being "extremely confident," how confident are you that you could exercise more?

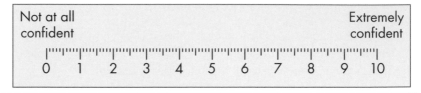

FIGURE 5–3.   Confidence ruler.

The same rules that apply with the importance ruler also apply with the confidence ruler. Resist the urge either to ask patients why they did not rate their confidence higher or to convince them that they are more confident than they perceive to be. Although natural to do so, these responses will likely trigger someone to find reasons to argue against your suggestions, which reinforces sustain talk. In order to avoid that pitfall, simply ask why the patient did not rate his or her confidence score lower. "You rated your confidence as a 3. Why didn't you rate it as a 1?" The patient's response will more than likely come in the form of change talk. If someone states 0, then ambivalence does not currently exist, and motivation is needed. "What would it take for it to go from 0 to 2?" As noted earlier for importance of change, this statement can be used anytime the patient does not have full confidence (10 on the confidence ruler).

Reviewing Past Successes

Simply reminding someone of past accomplishments can be helpful in unleashing hidden confidence. Most individuals have had to overcome a challenge at some point in their life. Reminding them of their ability to succeed is yet another avenue toward change. "You ran a 5K. How did you do that?" The more previous accomplishments are discussed, the more likely one's ability will be appreciated.

Using Hypotheticals

Speaking in hypotheticals allows for dialogue outside the realities of perceived restraints. Simply saying "What if…" provides freedom from limitations and allows for the formation of new thoughts ("What if you weren't so busy, how might you improve your diet?"). Removing the obstacle facilitates creativity, which can lead to a sense of empowerment in someone who lacks that sense of confidence.

Finding Motivation

These techniques are effective in someone actively contemplating change. However, if one has not contemplated such change, these techniques are less likely to be effective. Therefore, we should discuss how to evoke actual ambivalence.

Developing Discrepancy

Developing discrepancy can be a key component in unlocking motivation toward change. One develops this discrepancy through reality testing—evaluating thoughts by comparing them with real life. In real life, behavioral choices have consequences; highlighting those consequences leads one to engage in self-evaluation.

PATIENT: I always eat fast food.
CLINICIAN: You say your health is important; yet your diet seems not to reflect that.

Exchanging Information

Attempting to motivate someone by providing information can backfire if that information is already known. Therefore, it may be more advantageous to simply ask what is known first. In doing so, you can avoid providing redundant knowledge and address inaccuracies of thought, which may be the foundation of unhealthy choices.

PATIENT: I stopped taking the pills. They don't work.
CLINICIAN: What's your understanding of the medication?
PATIENT: I take them when I feel nervous…but I told you, it doesn't work.
CLINICIAN: May I provide you with some information about how the medication works?
PATIENT: Okay.
CLINICIAN: The medication needs time to work. The best results occur when taken daily for at least 4 weeks. I wasn't certain you were aware of that.
PATIENT: I didn't know that.
CLINICIAN: Now that you do, might you be willing to try the medication for at least 4 weeks?

Asking permission to give advice can minimize the likelihood of subsequent discord. Avoiding beginning your responses with "actually" can also decrease the perception of an adversarial exchange. After information is provided, interpretation can be elicited to better access likelihood of change.

Exploring Others' Concerns

Exploring the concerns of others is an excellent way to evoke motivation. Much like exchanging information, utilizing the perception of others can lower the likelihood of defensiveness and interpersonal discord.

CLINICIAN: What does your wife say about your drinking habits?
PATIENT: She says I drink too much and have gained weight.

These sorts of conversations can open a dialogue by identifying reasons for change. If an individual validates those reasons, then he or she has found merit in change.

EXAMPLE OF USE OF EVOKING IN MOTIVATIONAL INTERVIEWING

PATIENT: I have a hangover this morning.
CLINICIAN: You drank last night and now feel the effects this morning. [*Reflection*]
PATIENT: I drink every night, but usually I can hold my liquor.
CLINICIAN: Hangovers can be difficult to manage. [*Developing discrepancy*]
PATIENT: Yeah…today's been rough.
CLINICIAN: What did you used to do for fun before? [*Looking back*]
PATIENT: Well, I used to work out more.
CLINICIAN: Working out was enjoyable for you. [*Reflection*]
PATIENT: Yeah, I was going to the gym like every day.
CLINICIAN: It takes real commitment to work out every day. [*Affirmation*]
PATIENT: I don't think I could do that anymore.
CLINICIAN: Working out can be difficult when you have a hangover. [*Agreement with a twist*]
PATIENT: I don't always have a hangover. [*Interruption*]
CLINICIAN: I'm sorry to have implied that you're always hungover. I was wondering if you would work out more if you drank less. [*Apology, Redirection*]
PATIENT: Well…probably.
CLINICIAN: Is that something you'd like to do? [*Closed-ended evoking question*]
PATIENT: Well…yeah, I suppose. I don't really drink that much. [*Minimization*]
CLINICIAN: It seems you have the desire and ability to work out more. What are your thoughts about physical activity? [*Redirection, Open-ended evoking question*]
PATIENT: It's important. Heart disease runs in my family.
CLINICIAN: You've said that you want to work out more, have done so in the past, and it's important to you because of the family history of heart disease. [*Summary*]

KEY POINTS

- The mnemonic DARN CAT can be very helpful for remembering the various types of change talks:
  - Desire

  - Ability

  - Reasons

  - Need

  - Commitment

  - Activation

  - Taking steps

- The mnemonic OARS can be very helpful in remembering responsive skills that serve to reinforce and facilitate change talk:
  - Open questions
  - Affirmation
  - Reflection
  - Summaries
- Recognize
  - Ambivalence
  - Change talk (preparatory [DARN]/mobilizing [CAT])
  - Sustain talk (DARN CAT)
  - Discord (defensiveness, squaring off, interrupting, disengagement)
- Respond
  - Change talk (OARS)
  - Sustain talk (reflect and strategize)
  - Discord (reflect, strategize, apologize, affirm, redirect)
- Evoke
  - Change (questions, importance ruler, extremes, looking back/looking forward)
  - Confidence (talk, confidence ruler, review past successes, hypotheticals)
  - Motivation (discrepancy, exchanging information, others' concerns)
- Remembering acronyms and visualizing conceptual metaphors can aid in providing more salient memories of MI.
- The ruler is a conceptual metaphor that you can utilize to help evoke change talk. Imagine a ruler, which has been numbered 0 to 10. Next, ask the patient to rate the importance of change. Whatever number they report, ask them why a lower number was not chosen and reflect change talk. If the number is 0, then ask what it would take for the number to increase. The same technique can be used in evoking confidence.

STUDY QUESTIONS

1. Which evoking question is most likely to inspire change talk?

   A. Why are you drinking daily?
   B. Why not stop drinking?
   C. What are you thinking?
   D. What's the downside of drinking alcohol?

2. If you hear someone engaging in sustain talk, which of the following choices is the best response?

   A. Reframe.
   B. Affirm.
   C. Square off.
   D. Disengage.

3. Which of the following choices may worsen interpersonal discord?

   A. Apologize.
   B. Affirm.
   C. Square off.
   D. Redirect.

4. Which type of response is most likely to lead to sustain talk?

   A. Reflecting statement.
   B. Closed question.
   C. Affirmation.
   D. Summarizing statement.

5. Which of the following choices is an example of mobilizing change talk?

   A. Desire to change.
   B. Reasons to change.
   C. Ability to change.
   D. Commitment to change.

REFERENCES

Amrhein PC: The comprehension of quasi-performance verbs in verbal commitments: New evidence for componential theories of lexical meaning. Journal of Memory and Learning 31:756–784, 1992

Butler CC, Rollnick S, Cohen D, et al: Motivational consulting versus brief advice for smokers in general practice: a randomized trial. Br J Gen Pract 49(445):611–616, 1999

Miller WR, Rollnick S: Motivational Interviewing: Helping People Change, 3rd Edition. New York, Guilford, 2013

STUDENT REFLECTIONS

Anil Rengan
Rutgers New Jersey Medical School, MS-IV

The act of evoking motivation is paramount to initiating change in others. In order to do so, the medical interviewing process must be appreciated as a dynamic experience, a conversation during which various techniques are used to assess an individual's preparedness for making adjustments. By posing open-ended questions and hypotheticals, I allow patients the freedom to express themselves. The information provided, both verbal and nonverbal, is useful in identifying their level of ambivalence and stage of change. The initial encounter serves as a frame of reference for tracking a patient's progress, and the importance and confidence rulers are effective tools when reevaluating a patient's desire and ability to change throughout the process. Each step toward success should be commended through such techniques as affirmation, reflection, and reframing, regardless of how big or small the advancement. This instills confidence in patients and reminds them of the physician's supportive role.

I've often found myself at a loss for words when speaking with patients who firmly resist lifestyle modification. To counter this, perhaps I can try "agreeing with a twist" or attempt to redirect in a nonaccusatory manner. I should also be comfortable with apologizing if patients react defensively to my inquiries. With practice, these tactics will become more intuitive and spontaneous in nature.

An important facet of motivating patients is cementing the physician's position as a guiding light. As medical professionals, we must make patients aware that they are not alone, providing constant encouragement and assistance as they transform into healthier individuals.

Planning

Noah Capurso, M.D., M.H.S.

> A goal without a plan is just a wish.
>
> —*Antoine de Saint-Exupéry*

> By failing to prepare, you are preparing to fail.
>
> —*Benjamin Franklin*

> If you don't know where you are going, you'll end up someplace else.
>
> —*Yogi Berra*

The planning process of motivational interviewing (MI) transitions the patient from talking about change to conceiving a way toward implementing change. Successful and lasting change is more likely to be achieved if it is realized through the use of a carefully constructed plan. In the planning process, the clinician and patient collaboratively produce a clear step-by-step plan that the patient can execute in stages. This chapter presents strategies for recognizing when planning should take place, recommendations about how to productively collaborate on a plan, and components of successful change plans.

PLANNING AND MOTIVATIONAL INTERVIEWING

Planning is the fourth and final process of MI, along with engaging, focusing, and evoking, though the processes are not necessarily linear. During planning, the change talk that has been elicited throughout the other three processes is consolidated and transformed into a concrete step-by-step change plan. The change plan is the roadmap that guides the patient through the process of implementing change. The work of planning is to collaboratively construct a change plan that is both realistic and effective and then to support the patient through plan implementation. If setbacks are encountered along the way, as is often the case, revisiting the other three processes of MI can be helpful in supporting the process of change.

Of the four processes of MI, planning is the only one that is not always necessary when MI is properly being utilized. While MI requires that engaging, focusing, and evoking take place, patients will often initiate substantial changes on their own before formal planning ever begins. Occasionally, a patient may even achieve his or her ultimate goal, and the planning process becomes unnecessary. However, it is often the case that planning is an important and essential step toward helping patients achieve substantive and meaningful change.

Just as in the other three MI processes, maintaining a collaborative spirit throughout is key. The patient may continue to show signs of ambivalence, and continuing to listen for and evoke change talk remains a fundamental component of planning. Timing is also important. Shifting from evoking to planning at an appropriate time, when the patient shows the appropriate signs of readiness, maximizes the chances of successful change (Hettema et al. 2005). In fact, manualized MI protocols, in which the timing of progress from evoking to planning is standardized and inflexible, have been shown to be less effective than protocols that allow both patient and clinician to collaborate in deciding on the timing of this transition (Amrhein et al. 2003). A clinician (or patient) who jumps into planning prematurely risks lower chances of success.

TIMING OF PLANNING

Miller and Rollnick (2013) describe two ways to determine when a patient is ready to move from evoking to planning: *signs of readiness* and *testing the water.*

Assessing Signs of Readiness

In assessing signs of readiness, the clinician listens for and assesses both the frequency of individual change talk statements and the strength and nature of the statements themselves. The first clue in guiding the transition to planning may be the increased frequency of change talk. While listening to the patient, the clinician pays attention to preparatory change talk—statements that express desire, ability, reasons, and need to make a change (the DARN portion of the DARN CAT mnemonic), as well as mobilizing change talk statements that are assertions of commitment, activation, and taking steps (the CAT portion). Although both preparatory and mobilizing change talk are important forms of change talk, mobilizing change talk typically represents a stronger statement of change and is more indicative that a patient is readying for change. Therefore, the clinician should be sure to pay particular attention to mobilizing change talk statements.

Conversely, less frequent sustain talk is also a sign of the patient's readiness to progress to planning. A total cessation of sustain talk is unlikely. More typically, the clinician will begin to notice that a patient is approaching readiness for planning when the ratio of change talk to sustain talk begins to shift in favor of change. There is no defined threshold or percentage of change to sustain talk that absolutely indicates whether a patient is truly ready to begin formulating a change plan. It will be up to the clinician's judgment as to when this balance has been reached. Taking each individual patient's style and ways of talking about change into account will be important in assessing readiness to change.

Another clue that the patient is readying for planning is that he or she will begin to imagine a future in which the change he or she desires has been achieved. The patient may begin to ask questions of a practical nature that reflect both hopes and concerns about postchange life. For example, a patient who is trying to stop drinking might ask a hopeful practical question such as "How much money do you think I will save if I wasn't buying alcohol?" On the other hand, the patient might express concern in a question such as "What will I do when I watch the game with my friends when all of them drink?" Both of these types of questions are encouraging. While the latter question may sound like sustain talk, it is a sign that the patient is beginning to sort through the day-to-day aspects of what achieving and maintaining change might mean for his or her lifestyle.

Similarly, patients ready to change will begin asking questions of a very practical nature about how change might be accomplished. The more concrete or even mundane the question, the more likely it is that the patient is ready to begin planning and subsequently take steps toward change. For instance, a general question such as "Do you think I will feel better when I quit smoking?" is less indicative of a readiness for change than a specific question such as "What are the locations of some stores where I can buy nicotine gum?" Both questions signify that the patient is thinking about quitting, but the specifics of that latter question indicate that the person not only is thinking about quitting but is curious about a particular strategy, nicotine replacement, and would like to know about how to take steps toward implementing that strategy.

Finally, patients ready for planning often have begun to take small steps toward action on their own. Perhaps they have made efforts to stop smoking in the house or have already started substituting nicotine gum for some cigarettes if their goal is to quit smoking. Someone trying to stop drinking excessively may alternate alcoholic drinks with nonalcoholic ones or switch to drinks with lower alcohol content. These steps show that the patient is already beginning to formulate and act on a change plan. Regardless of the specifics, it's helpful to notice such actions and affirm that they are steps toward change.

Signs of readiness to listen for

- Preparatory change talk
- Mobilizing change talk
- Decreasing strength and frequency of sustain talk
- Practical questions about how to achieve change
- Practical questions about a postchange future
- Taking small steps toward change

Testing the Water

When you feel that all signs point to the patient's readiness to begin formal planning, it can be helpful to assess the degree of readiness and set the stage for the transition by testing the water. This is achieved by summarizing the content of all the change talk heard thus far, presenting the summary to the patient, and then posing a key question about how the patient would like to proceed next. The patient's response to this key question will likely serve as an indicator as to whether he or she is ready for planning.

The summary statement, or recapitulation, should consist of all the compelling change talk made by the patient over the course of the entire therapy. Inclusion of sustain talk or other reasons to resist change should be avoided in the summary statement, whenever possible. The goal is to present all the arguments the patient has made for change. The statement can be a means of gaining perspective on the progress made thus far, as well as serve as a reminder to the patient of any important change talk that might have been forgotten. The summary statement can be conceptualized as a curated "bouquet" of change talk collected throughout the sessions by the clinician, with each stem representing a reason supporting change.

Following the delivery of the summary statement, it can be useful to pause in order to allow the patient to digest the contents just presented, and then pose a key question about how the patient would best like to proceed. The placement of the key question immediately following the presentation of all the reasons to change is important; it sets the stage for change and opens the door for the patient to say that he or she wants to start making concrete and substantial progress toward change. It also leaves open the possibility that the patient is not yet quite ready for planning and invites him or her to reflect on that possibility as well.

Example of testing the water

Testing the water for a patient trying to quit smoking might go like this:

> You have made some compelling arguments for quitting smoking over the course of our working together. You mentioned that your doctor has warned you that quitting smoking is critical for your health because you are beginning to develop chronic obstructive pulmonary disease; you do not want to ever depend upon an oxygen tank. Your family frequently nags you to quit, which you find annoying and frustrating, as well as embarrassing at large family gatherings. Finally, the financial costs of smoking have become burdensome as the price of cigarettes continues to increase. As you mentioned last time, you spend more on cigarettes than on your car payments each month. You have already cut down from a pack and a half to a pack a day and say that you are committed to quitting for good.

This is the time to pause for a few seconds in order to allow the patient to sit with all this change talk, presented together, and think about its implications. After the pause, the clinician may ask the key question:

> Given all this, how do you think you would like to proceed from here?"

If the patient indicates in the answer to the key question that he or she would like to continue toward his or her change goal, it's time to begin formally developing a change plan.

CHANGE PLANNING

A change plan is a roadmap, collaboratively created between patient and clinician, that lays out the step-by-step process by which the ultimate change goal can be achieved. There are specific features of change plans that optimize chances of success, and ways to go about creating such change plans (as described later in this chapter), but regardless of the specific features and methods, it is important that the clinician maintain the open and accepting spirit of MI throughout the planning process.

Listening for Change Talk

The best change plans consist primarily of strategies that originate with the patient. The clinician may, with permission, make suggestions, but it is the patient who should be considered the expert on himself or herself and, consequently, the person best equipped to predict which strategies are most likely to lead to success. Therefore, it is especially important to listen for change talk that mentions specific actions and abilities. For instance, a patient trying to stay sober from cocaine may say, "I could delete the numbers of all the dealers I know from my phone—that way I won't be able to call them and get cocaine when I feel a craving." The clinician is encouraged to remind the patient of such statements later during the change planning; it is through such specific and mobilizing change talk that an effective change plan is built.

Although the task of the clinician is to elicit a change plan consisting of strategies that originate with the patient, it is useful to guide the planning process toward steps that are relatively small and clear. The more specific the components of the change plan, the better. A statement such as "I will smoke two less cigarettes each day for the next 5 days" is more likely to lead to change than "I will cut down some on the amount I smoke over the next several days." Such statements of intention are more likely to lead to success if the plan is specific and has a clear method of implementation (Gollwitzer 1999).

Setting SMART Goals

A useful framework to utilize in the development of a change plan is the concept of SMART goals (Table 6–1). SMART goals have been used in various fields of medicine and business in the development of clear goals designed to foster change (Bovend'Eerdt et al. 2009). SMART stands for specific, measurable, action-oriented, realistic, and time-bound. There are literally dozens of variations of the SMART mnemonic (Rubin 2002)—the one presented here is just one among many—however, they all encapsulate the same concept; a goal should be specific and quantifiable, so that whether or not the goal has been achieved can be mutually agreed on by clinician and patient.

The goal should be achievable through some type of action and should be realistic in the sense that it is achievable, allowing for success rather than unrealistic and increasing the likelihood of failure. Finally, the goal should have a predetermined time limit at which point the clinician and patient can come together and determine whether or not the goal was achieved.

It's still possible to capitalize on a vague statement like the one given above (i.e., "I will cut down some on the amount I smoke over the next several days"). Such a statement still constitutes change talk and can certainly be used to move the process of planning forward. At this point, praise for the patient's commitment to change is due. The goal can then be refined and made "SMARTer"

TABLE 6–1.	Some variations of the SMART mnemonic (adapted from Rubin 2002)

S—specific, simple, significant

M—measurable, meaningful, motivating

A—action-oriented, actionable, acceptable, achievable, accountable, agreed-upon, assignable

R—realistic, reviewable, rewarding, results-oriented, relevant to a mission

T—time-bound, tangible, timely, time-based, timed, toward what you want, truthful

through further collaborative work with the patient. Possible follow-up questions may be "How many cigarettes do you think you might be able to cut out?" and "When might we look back and see whether or not you were able to meet your goal?"

Example of a SMART goal

"I will smoke two less cigarettes each day for the next 5 days."

- Specific: focus on smoking cigarettes
- Measurable: two cigarettes daily
- Action-oriented: abstaining from smoking
- Realistic: this depends on the patient's circumstances
- Time-bound: reassessed in 5 days

Emphasizing Change Planning and Collaboration

Sometimes, patients will have developed a change plan on their own before the planning process formally commences during therapy. For instance, patients trying to cut down or abstain from alcohol may already have had a period of sobriety in the past. Smokers may have been able to quit before. In these cases, using the tried-and-true strategy to achieve sobriety may be the best way to proceed. Honing specifics of the plan and keeping them consistent with the principles of SMART goals can be helpful. The clinician's role under these circumstances is to support the patient to implement the plan.

More commonly, the patient will have some ideas as to how to proceed without a fully formed change plan ready to implement, and there will be several viable paths forward. In this case, the clinician's role is to winnow down the options. Clarifying the ultimate end goal, determining whether there are smaller subgoals to aim for along the way, and prioritizing the options, called *path mapping*, can be helpful in this task (Miller and Rollnick 2013).

Information and advice

Change planning should be a collaborative process. However, a clinician can still provide information and advice to the patient as long as it is done in a manner consistent with the spirit of MI. To ensure that the information or advice is welcome, it is important that the clinician have permission to make the offer. Permission can be given either implicitly (the patient asks for it) or explicitly (the clinician asks, "Is it okay if I offer you some advice?").

For instance, a patient who abuses alcohol may have an ultimate goal of complete sobriety, but he or she may not quite know where to start. The patient may be wondering whether the first step should consist of cutting back gradually, or cutting down significantly, or stopping altogether. Moreover, the patient may be questioning whether to use medication or psychosocial interventions alone. He or she may have heard different reports of how participation in support groups such as Alcoholic Anonymous compares with individualized treatment in a medical setting. It is likely that such a patient will be contemplating all these options simultaneously.

The goal is not to tell the patient what the patient *should* do, but rather to explore the pros and cons of each option in the eyes of the patient. Does the patient have any hunches about where to start? What are the patient's preferences? The clinician and patient can create an ordered list of the options, designating which plan to start with, and specifying where the patient might go if the plan does not succeed.

Sometimes, the patient will have no idea about how to achieve change. Patients who abuse substances and have never had a period of sobriety may not know of any first steps toward abstinence. At other times, the clinician may not know of a clear path forward either. For instance, substances of abuse such as new designer drugs do not have treatments that have a broad base of supporting evidence. In this scenario, the clinician and patient can brainstorm various change plan options collaboratively. The clinician can offer information and advice and generate ideas with the patient, as long as permission is given. Once a list of options is generated, the options can be ordered and the first-choice option can be determined (Table 6–2).

Once a change plan is finalized, it is important to ensure that the patient understands the details of each step, especially if planning has stretched out over

TABLE 6–2.   Change planning and collaboration

IF	Patient has a formulated plan	Patient has some ideas for a plan	Patient has no ideas where to begin
THEN	Provide support Hone specifics Keep goals consistent with SMART	Use path mapping Clarify end goal Explore pros and cons of each option	Collaboratively brainstorm Offer advice with permission

multiple sessions. Going back over the plan step by step to serve as a reminder of its components can be useful. It is critical that the plan be discussed explicitly so that the patient can appreciate the context of each step and the path forward (Tevyaw and Monti 2004).

PERSISTING THROUGH CHANGE

Even during planning and implementation, as the patient makes progress toward his or her change goal, it is natural and normal for commitment to waver. Relapse to substance use or slower-than-expected progress toward sobriety could prove discouraging. It is at times of flagging commitment that the clinician takes the opportunity to strengthen commitment, with the goal of transforming motivation into commitment and commitment into action toward change.

Understanding Implementation Intentions

It is important that a clinician continue to support and promote mobilizing change talk. Ideally, in the course of treatment the patient will express what is termed an *implementation intention*—a particularly potent form of mobilizing change talk that is associated with change success. An implementation intention statement consists of two components: an expression of intent to complete a specific action and an expression of that intent to another person (Gollwitzer 1999; Rise et al. 2003). The inclusion of another person in the content of the implementation intention invokes the assistance of another and holds the person making the intention responsible not only to themselves but to someone else as well.

An example of a strong implementation intention is "Yes doctor, I will smoke five less cigarettes each day for the next week until our next appointment." It consists of a specific action (cutting down on smoking) with a commitment directed toward another person (the doctor). In MI, the most common other person is the clinician; however, the implementation intention can be equally or even more powerful if the other person invoked is a loved one—for example, "I will promise my wife that I will drink no more than two drinks a day." The inclusion of the patient's wife is an indicator that the wife will act as a support for the patient through the process of change and will also hold the patient responsible for his or her actions.

Implementation intention

A particularly potent form of change talk consisting of two parts:

- A specific action
- Direction toward a specific person

Example: "Yes doctor, I will smoke five less cigarettes each day for the next week until our next appointment."

It should be kept in mind, however, that while mobilizing change talk is associated with improved chances of success in reaching a change goal, and efforts should be made to promote it, change can still be achieved in the absence of mobilizing change talk. Preparatory change talk alone has been associated with achieving change (Baer et al. 2008). It is the underlying process of all change talk, motivation, which is the necessary ingredient for change.

Breaking Down Change Plans: Stepping-Stones

One technique for promoting mobilizing change talk in a patient with diminishing commitment is to break down the change plan into smaller, more achievable goals. A patient who is feeling demoralized following a return to drinking is more likely to be able to commit to the statement "I will not drink today" than to a larger, more distant goal such as "I will stop drinking completely."

Small change goals and ways to support change can be customized to the patient's commitment. For example, the patient willing to commit to not drinking one day at a time may also be able to commit to taking disulfiram in the morning, again, one day at a time. A patient considering participation in Alcoholics Anonymous may feel overwhelmed committing to 90 meetings in 90 days (a common goal following an alcohol relapse) but may be willing to commit to three meetings in the next week or even one meeting *today*.

When the clinician is presenting the concept of breaking down a change plan into smaller, achievable pieces, a useful metaphor can be that of *stepping-stones*. The process of change can be thought of as a wide river—the more difficult the change, the wider the river. The patient's goal is to ultimately reach the opposite shore. A change plan of quitting smoking or drinking alcohol all at once is analogous to a change plan of trying to make it across the river in a single bound. Multiple failed attempts at trying to clear the river this way would be disheartening in addition to being unrealistic. Breaking an ultimate goal down into smaller pieces is placing stepping-stones across the river—each intermediate goal represents a single stepping-stone. The wider the river, the more stepping-stones will be required, with each one taking the patient closer to his or her goal of reaching the other side.

Seemingly small commitments can be strikingly effective at achieving change. For example, having patients monitor their own substance use is an intervention that many patients will agree to as an initial step in their change plan, yet this simple act of record keeping can help cut down on use. Heavy drinkers who began keeping track of the number of drinks consumed before each drink were shown to reduce their consumption by as much as one-third (Miller et al. 1980). Perhaps the patient would be willing to tell a loved one about his or her commitment to change; enlisting the support of a close social contact has been shown to decrease drinking behaviors as well (Barber and Crisp 1995).

These two approaches can be combined into a strategy termed *supportive monitoring*, in which, in the case of drinking, a loved one keeps track of the patient's drinking behavior. The most important source of ideas for the change plan is the patient; however, these strategies can be suggested, with permission, for the patient who would benefit from small yet meaningful steps on the road to the ultimate change goal.

IMPLEMENTATION OF A CHANGE PLAN

MI is often seen as a way of initial engagement—a way to help patients invest in the idea of making a change. However, MI can be useful throughout the implementation of a change plan.

It is important for both clinician and patient to appreciate that the path toward permanent and lasting change is often not linear. Acknowledging that setbacks are a normal part of recovery can help prevent patients from getting discouraged and providers from getting burned out. Not reaching set goals, waning motivation, resumption of substance use after a period of sobriety, and other setbacks are common. A patient dropping out of treatment and re-presenting for treatment after some time, particularly following a setback, is common as well.

For many patients, substance use has become an integral part of their lives, and for them sobriety requires not only abstinence but a shift in lifestyle as well. Patients often continue to require support as they implement change plans and especially if unforeseen roadblocks present. Similar to substance abuse, conditions such as depression and anxiety often tend to reappear at times of particular stress. These situations can be addressed in a manner similar to substance abuse.

Continuing regular meetings as the patient implements his or her change plan can be useful in catching setbacks early. Whether the setback is increasing substance use, falling behind on meeting scheduled goals, or even just waning motivation, catching setbacks early allows them to be addressed directly and worked through before they grow into something larger. Normalizing setbacks and presenting them as part of the change process can be helpful in maintaining morale and can prevent a change plan from being entirely derailed.

Revisiting Other Motivational Interviewing Processes

Just as a patient's journey toward change is often not linear, the processes of MI do not necessarily have to be sequential. Focusing builds on engaging, evoking builds on focusing, and planning builds on evoking; however, revisiting the other processes during the planning stage, or even as a change plan is being implemented, can prove useful.

Planning

A common process to revisit is to take just a single step back and return to planning. Revisiting planning can be especially useful after the patient encounters a setback or finds that the original change plan is not working. A return to planning following a setback can be especially useful because the nature of the setback and the shortcomings of the previous plan can be examined. Simply asking the patient "What else?" or "What now?" can serve as a segue and invitation back into the process of planning.

Evoking (or "Reminding")

Returning to the process of evoking, called "reminding" by Miller and Rollnick (2013), is valuable for the patient whose commitment or motivation is wavering. Frequent setbacks or simply pursuing a goal for a prolonged period of time can exhaust a patient's commitment. Wavering commitment can lead to diminishing interest or investment in making change. Oftentimes, a brief return to evoking can serve as a reminder as to the reasons why the patient is trying to make a change in the first place. Simply exploring a patient's commitment with a comment like "Tell me about the importance of achieving this goal" can trigger the change talk necessary to strengthen motivation to change.

Focusing

Sometimes, a patient may change his or her desired goal midcourse during the process of change. Perhaps a smoker who originally wanted to cut down to less than half a pack per day has been doing so well that the new goal becomes quitting completely. Perhaps a patient with an opiate use disorder whose goal was to stop opiate use without the assistance of medications has been having such a difficult time that the new goal becomes transitioning onto a maintenance medication such as methadone. A patient trying to lose weight might change his or her target weight depending on how difficult implementing the plan has been for him or her.

Such course corrections are common and can be a natural part of the change process. It is in these times that it is helpful to return to focusing. An exploration of the patient's priorities, preferences, and values can be revisited. Efforts are then made to define the new goal explicitly, and, once defined, a change plan can be collaboratively created.

Engaging

Some patients may begin to question whether making change is worth the effort at all. The patient can become disengaged, and without engagement, it is difficult to persist on the path to change. Once a patient becomes progressively disengaged, getting him or her to reinvest the time and energy into making change can be difficult. Disengagement often manifests as a return to substance use.

It is therefore prudent to catch signs of disengagement as early as possible. Eliciting feedback at the end of each session can be helpful in identifying early disengagement. Following up after the conclusion of therapy with a phone call can also help the clinician catch signs of disengagement, hopefully before it leads to a return to substance use.

Any signs of disengagement, such as missing appointments, arriving late, and not implementing steps agreed on during previous sessions, should be addressed directly. Just as in engaging, reengaging consists of posing open questions, affirmations, reflections, and summaries (referred to as OARS). Revisiting the process of engaging with the patient who seems to be actively disengaging can be crucial in preventing the loss of any progress (Table 6–3).

Avoiding Pejorative Language

The language used to frame the process of change is important. The lexicon of addiction is full of pejorative terms that are antithetical to the spirit of MI; such terms are best avoided. Using a label for the patient such as "addict," "alcoholic," or "user" is demeaning and denies the complexity of the patient suffering with addiction. Another commonly used example is the word "relapse." This term suggests that the process of recovery consists of only two states, abstinence and relapse; use of the term dismisses any appreciation of the spectrum of use patterns. It does not support a patient who has been able to cut down, and it does not distinguish between 1 drink and 20.

Such dichotomous thinking can be discouraging, especially for the patient who often continues a level of use during the process of recovery. Patients who conceptualize any substance use as a "relapse" may give up on their change plan after using even a small amount of substance because they view themselves as having relapsed and therefore having failed treatment, a phenomenon termed the *abstinence violation effect* (Curry et al. 1987).

TABLE 6–3.	When to revisit the four processes of motivational interviewing
Replanning	Small setbacks in the original change plan
	Need for smaller, more discrete change steps
Reevoking	Wavering commitment
	Frequent setbacks
	Diminishing interest
Refocusing	Desire for a new change goal—"course correction"
Reengaging	Loss of interest
	Return to substance abuse
	Frequent missed appointments/late arrivals

Using Motivational Interviewing as a Complementary Tool

Finally, MI is not to be used in isolation. The spirit of MI, as well as various components of MI, can be freely combined and integrated with other psychotherapeutic and pharmacological approaches at the discretion of the clinician. Combination therapies have been evaluated extensively in the literature, with clinical trials conducted combining aspects of MI with many other modalities.

MI may be particularly useful when combined with cognitive-behavioral therapy (CBT), especially during planning. MI focuses on the "why" of change, and CBT focuses on "how" that change might be achieved. The tools afforded by CBT may be helpful in laying out a concrete step-by-step change plan. Combining MI with other treatment approaches will be covered in detail in Chapter 7 ("Integrating Motivational Interviewing With Other Psychotherapies") and Chapter 8 ("Motivational Interviewing and Pharmacotherapy").

EXAMPLES OF USE OF PLANNING IN MOTIVATIONAL INTERVIEWING

Testing the Water: Recapitulation and Key Question (Drinking)

> CLINICIAN: We've had several meetings where we discussed your feelings about cutting down and possibly eventually stopping drinking.
> PATIENT: That's right. I've been thinking about it for a while. It's gotten to the point that I really need to at least dial it back a bit.
> CLINICIAN: You're thinking that it is time for a change.

PATIENT: Yes, I think I need to do something. I can't go on like this.

CLINICIAN: You're ready to make a change. I'd like to offer you a summary of what we've discussed to make sure that we're both on the same page. Then we call talk about how best to proceed. How does that sound?

PATIENT: Yes, that sounds good.

CLINICIAN: Thank you for all that you have shared with me. You've been running into trouble with drinking for quite a few years at this point. Blackouts at the end of nights of drinking are scary for you, and you've gotten into some altercations that certainly could have been avoided if you were sober. There haven't been any legal problems yet, but you've driven while intoxicated on multiple occasions and you worry about getting into an accident, hurting someone, or even getting arrested. You've also noticed that your cravings for alcohol have only gotten stronger, and recently you've been getting nervous and even a little shaky when you go for more than a day without any alcohol. Finally, it was a tipping point for you to seek treatment when your doctor said your high blood pressure is likely due to drinking. The fact that several of your family members have had heart problems makes you especially worried. You are thinking of cutting down on your drinking and are curious to explore options for achieving that. (*Pause*) So, where would you like to go from here?

PATIENT: Yeah, that's all true. I'm not sure exactly where to go, but, as you said, I definitely want to cut back on my drinking.

CLINICIAN: Well, if it's okay with you, we could start talking about some specific strategies to construct a change plan based on what you've mentioned thus far.

PATIENT: That sounds good. I'd be interested in that.

Setting a SMART Goal (Smoking)

CLINICIAN: You've told me of your commitment to stop smoking. Quitting cold turkey hasn't worked for you in the past, and it's oftentimes useful to set some intermediate goals along the way. How would you like to proceed today?

PATIENT: We could try having some smaller goals. How about if I cut down some on the amount I smoke over the next several days? I could come in and tell you how much I was able to cut down when I come in next week.

CLINICIAN: That's a great start. It's good you want to cut down over the next week, and we can make that a little bit more specific. How many cigarettes do you think you want to start eliminating per day?

PATIENT: I'm not sure. I smoke a pack and a half every day right now. It would probably be easiest if I cut out a few each day. What do you think?

CLINICIAN: I think that sounds like a good idea. So if you were to cut out a few cigarettes every day, how many would you want to cut out?

PATIENT: Two? I think I'd be able to do that.

CLINICIAN: Great. Your goal is to cut down by two cigarettes each day.

PATIENT: Yeah, that sounds doable. It's not too big of a change but it will certainly add up. Actually, now that I think about it, that would mean I would be smoking 10 cigarettes less after 5 days. That's half a pack!

CLINICIAN: That's right. When you think about it that way, what do you think about the plan?

PATIENT: I'd say that 10 cigarettes is probably a good goal for the first week. I doubt I could do more than that. How about this? I'll smoke two less cigarettes each day for the next 5 days. That'll get me down to one pack a day, and I'll try to maintain it at that level until we meet a week from today.

CLINICIAN: Well, we have a plan then. Let's meet next week and check in.

KEY POINTS

When Should Planning Begin?

- *Signs of readiness:* increased ratio of change to sustain talk, strengthening change talk statements, planning for change.

- *Testing the water:* present a "bouquet" of change talk (recapitulation); ask the key question "What would you like to do next?"

Creating a Robust Change Plan

- The best plans are clear and precise.

- SMART Goals: specific, measurable, action-oriented, realistic, and time-bound. Change planning should remain collaborative—maintain the motivational interviewing (MI) spirit.

If Commitment Diminishes

- Remember that fluctuating commitment is normal in the process of change.

- Listen for and support any residual mobilizing change talk.

- Ask, "What else might help you commit to your change goal?"

- Break the change plan down into smaller, more achievable steps.

- Consider useful suggestions (with permission) such as self-monitoring and enlisting the support of a significant other.

As the Plan Is Being Implemented

- Support the change being made (this is essential).

- Avoid pejorative language and dichotomous ("black and white") thinking about goals.

- Encourage: catch setbacks early and normalize the nonlinear nature of change.

- Consider revisiting the other MI processes in supporting change.

Remember that MI can be integrated with other therapeutic approaches.

STUDY QUESTIONS

1. You've been working with a patient to cut down on drinking for the past 2 months. Recently, he has been late to appointments and has canceled a few times. When you do meet, he reveals that his drinking has been increasing. What stage of motivational interviewing (MI) is the most appropriate to revisit at this time?

     A. Replanning.
     B. Reevoking ("reminding").
     C. Refocusing.
     D. Reengaging.
     E. None; this patient's care should be transferred to another clinician.

2. *Recapitulation* refers to

     A. Repeating the patient's change talk back to them verbatim.
     B. Mirroring the patient's body language.
     C. Making a summary statement of collected change talk.
     D. One of the four fundamental processes of MI.
     E. The process of creating a change plan.

3. The "SMART" in SMART goals can stand for

     A. Sensible, maintainable, attune, resistance, two-part.
     B. Specific, measurable, action-oriented, realistic, time-bound.
     C. Serviceable, multiple, attached, richly developed, traditional.
     D. Stages, most-rewarding, autonomous, referenced, tolerable.
     E. Support, mindful, accurate, responsible, theoretical.

4. Your patient is in the process of implementing a well-designed change plan but is having trouble achieving the goals she has set for herself. What might be the most useful next step?

     A. Advise her on strategies that you think might be helpful.
     B. Tell her that she needs to make a more sustained effort.
     C. Break down the change plan into smaller, more achievable intermediate goals.
     D. Be realistic and realize that she probably will not be able to achieve lasting change; helping her come to terms with this now will minimize disappointment in the end.
     E. Introduce her to another patient who achieved a similar goal.

5. Which of the following statements represents mobilizing change talk for a patient trying to quit smoking?

    A. "I bought a box of nicotine patches yesterday and put one on for the first time this morning."

    B. "The cravings for cigarettes can be so powerful sometimes."

    C. "I know that smoking is bad for my health."

    D. "My family is always giving me a hard time about smoking. I really hope that I'm able to kick this habit!"

    E. "I could buy a car with the amount of money I spend on cigarettes."

REFERENCES

Amrhein PC, Miller WR, Yahne CE, et al: Client commitment language during motivational interviewing predicts drug use outcomes. J Consult Clin Psychol 71(5):862–878, 2003 14516235

Baer JS, Beadnell B, Garrett SB, et al: Adolescent change language within a brief motivational intervention and substance use outcomes. Psychol Addict Behav 22(4):570–575, 2008 19071983

Barber JG, Crisp BR: Social support and prevention of relapse following treatment for alcohol abuse. Research on Social Work Practice 5:283–296, 1995

Bovend'Eerdt TJ, Botell RE, Wade DT: Writing SMART rehabilitation goals and achieving goal attainment scaling: a practical guide. Clin Rehabil 23(4):352–361, 2009 19237435

Curry S, Marlatt GA, Gordon JR: Abstinence violation effect: validation of an attributional construct with smoking cessation. J Consult Clin Psychol 55(2):145–149, 1987 3571666

Gollwitzer P: Implementation intentions: strong effects of simple plans. Am Psychol 54:493–503, 1999

Hettema J, Steele J, Miller WR: Motivational interviewing. Annu Rev Clin Psychol 1:91–111, 2005 17716083

Miller WR, Rollnick S: Motivational Interviewing: Helping People Change, 3rd Edition. New York, Guilford, 2013

Miller WR, Taylor CA, West JC: Focused versus broad-spectrum behavior therapy for problem drinkers. J Consult Clin Psychol 48(5):590–601, 1980 7410657

Rise J, Thompson M, Verplanken B: Measuring implementation intentions in the context of the theory of planned behavior. Scand J Psychol 44(2):87–95, 2003 12778976

Rubin RS: Will the real SMART goals please stand up? Ind Organ Psychol 39(4):26–27, 2002

Tevyaw TO, Monti PM: Motivational enhancement and other brief interventions for adolescent substance abuse: foundations, applications and evaluations. Addiction 99(suppl 2):63–75, 2004 15488106

STUDENT REFLECTIONS

Amy Schettino
Yale School of Medicine, MS3

The planning stage of motivational interviewing (MI), while not necessary in some patients, can be a critical step in achieving true change in others. Always assess the patient's readiness to progress by summarizing their "change talk" and offering the option of moving forward. When creating the plan, remember to keep it a collaborative process, reminding the patient of his or her own earlier suggestions or discussing the pros and cons of several options. Ensure the patient verbalizes his or her plan, step by step, to you or a significant other, and keep an eye out for signs of disengagement. If the patient becomes discouraged, it can be helpful to set smaller goals and normalize relapse or slow progress.

While planning often occurs after several sessions and a long-standing relationship with the patient, it also has applications in fields where patient contact is comparatively brief, such as inpatient medicine. As a medical student, I have time to sit down with patients and discuss the risk factors and causes behind their hospitalization. These conversations are often a great time for planning with the patient, and I may be able to help the patient decide on what action to take before his or her next follow-up appointment. For instance, I could suggest 20 minutes of walking per day, only drinking soda twice per week, or beginning group therapy for addiction or depression. If the patient already has a plan but became discouraged, I have the opportunity to refocus his or her efforts toward achievable goals. In the hospital, the patient's illness is a new and present motivator and may lend extra strength to your interview and the rewards of enacting change.

Getting Good at Motivational Interviewing

Integrating Motivational Interviewing With Other Psychotherapies

Marie-Josée Lynch, M.D., C.M.

Bachaar Arnaout, M.D.

Richard N. Rosenthal, M.D.

> If I am at all successful, I would hope to be read somewhat mythically, that is, less concerned with literal issues than with conveying the larger melody of change.
>
> —*Edgar A. Levenson*

An important question that often arises when working from a motivational interviewing (MI) stance is whether MI can be woven into other forms of psychotherapy. There is a menu of psychotherapeutic treatment options for patients with substance use disorders, one of the most common indications for MI (Najavits and Weiss 1994). MI is compatible with many of these therapeutic modalities (Miller and Rollnick 2013), and combining MI with other psychotherapies not only enhances the efficacy of both treatments but also sustains the MI effect (Hettema et al. 2005). Intuitively, one would expect the importance of MI to be at its peak early in the process of engaging in treatment, when patients are often still contemplative about addressing their substance use or other behavioral goals (see, e.g., Brady et al. 2001). Accordingly, MI has often been described as a "prelude" to other interventions. It is important to underline that MI need not be abandoned once a patient has mustered sufficient motivation to move forward and engage in treatment. Motivation is a fluid phenomenon, and its strength inevitably fluctuates. A skilled therapist is able to use MI in a manner that is tailored to the individual patient's needs by continuing to assess progress through a motivational lens. This allows for the selective reintroduction of MI principles at therapeutic choice points when ambivalence resurfaces.

It is helpful to have a sense of how the different therapeutic components of the recovery journey can mesh together when working with a patient. From a training perspective, different psychotherapeutic approaches are typically taught separately, with little consideration of how they can be used jointly to provide a more customized treatment. This conflicts with the practice of psychotherapy, which typically transcends the boundaries set by training programs and treatment manuals. One can argue that strict adherence to a rigid therapeutic approach serves to treat the therapist more than the patient, because it can be intimidating to conceptualize how the many different pieces of the therapeutic arsenal can fit together. Therapeutic flexibility is an essential asset for modern, patient-centered treatment, because patients often have multiple comorbidities and stand to benefit from a variety of modalities. The patient's needs change dynamically throughout the course of therapy, and one must be able to adjust the approach to match the patient's goals. No treatment is a panacea. At the same time, eclecticism poses theoretical and practical challenges and may render psychotherapy unfocused, or perhaps less effective, at times. Our aim in this chapter is to share some practical ways to integrate MI with other common psychotherapeutic modalities, while mindful of the pitfalls of haphazard eclecticism.

INTEGRATIVE PSYCHOTHERAPY THEORY

Types of Psychotherapy Integration

Integrated approaches to psychotherapy have been gaining in popularity, and a literature exists describing strategies to weave together elements from different psychotherapeutic schools of thought. Four major types of psychotherapy integration have been elaborated: theoretical integration, assimilative integration, technical eclecticism, and the common factors approach (Stricker and Gold 1996). *Theoretical integration* seeks to generate new theories composed of elements of two or more established schools of thought. This approach is by far the most complex and, consequently, the least practical for the purposes of this text. It will, therefore, not be discussed further here. *Assimilative integration* involves using the framework of one particular approach, while bringing in elements of another modality, as clinically indicated. *Technical eclecticism*—a variant of assimilative integration—involves the sequencing of two or more psychotherapeutic approaches in a manner that is tailored to the patient's needs, without a primary grounding theoretical base. Finally, the *common factors approach* postulates that effective therapies share common active ingredients, and it endeavors to maximize their use. Carl Rogers was a proponent of the common factors approach, and his writings focused on how personal growth can be catalyzed by therapists who demonstrate accurate empathy, unconditional positive regard, and self-congruence, which serve to enhance the quality of the therapeutic relationship (Rogers 1957). These common factors are deemed vital irrespective of the psychotherapeutic modality. They also resonate with the core elements of the spirit of MI, which is rooted in the Rogerian client-centered approach (Miller and Rollnick 2013).

Sequenced Versus Combined Approaches to Psychotherapy Integration

For the purposes of this chapter, the therapy integration theories will be separated into two categories: sequenced approaches and combined approaches. A *sequenced* approach consists of using two or more psychotherapy techniques in their pure form in an alternating manner to match patient need. Assimilative integration and technical eclecticism belong to this category. Sequenced approaches to integrating MI are particularly useful when the challenge of ambivalence rears its head. A common example is the use of an interlude of MI during the course of cognitive-behavioral therapy (CBT) when the patient is demonstrating ambivalence about the treatment (which often manifests as challenges with homework completion). Changing therapeutic gears allows MI to be delivered with the goal of resolving ambivalence about engaging in the therapy. Further examples of this approach will be explored in this chapter.

Combined approaches, such as the common factors approach, simultaneously use elements of two therapies to form a synergistic whole. As a guiding principle, one can employ combined approaches to enhance the therapeutic alliance. Blending of core MI principles within another psychotherapeutic framework serves to boost the therapeutic relationship on which the work of therapy can unfold. The appropriateness of this integration technique depends on the compatibility between the two theories being united.

In this chapter, we use these general principles to help guide a discussion of the ways in which MI can be integrated into other commonly used psychotherapy modalities in the treatment of substance use disorders. More specifically, CBT, psychodynamic therapy, supportive psychotherapy, and group therapy will be explored, and practical tips will be provided to guide the design of integrated treatment plans.

MOTIVATIONAL INTERVIEWING AND COGNITIVE-BEHAVIORAL THERAPY

CBT is widely recognized as a first-line psychotherapy in the treatment of addictive disorders (Carroll and Onken 2005). Its use in this field is based on social learning theory, which posits that substance use is a learned behavior that is perpetuated by operant conditioning, such that the pairing of alcohol or drugs with conditioned stimuli serves to maintain their use. Conditioned stimuli can consist of objects, people, situations, or internal states. A common example of such paired stimuli is the association between coffee and cigarettes, whose mutual reinforcement may make coffee a particularly potent trigger for individuals attempting to quit smoking.

CBT for substance use disorders can be divided into two main components. The first consists of a *functional analysis of substance use*, which entails a close inquiry into the patient's typical pattern of use, with particular attention paid to the antecedents and consequences of using. This analysis allows for the identification of common triggers for use and assists in predicting which situations are high-risk. Once these high-risk conditions are identified, the focus of therapy becomes the acquisition of coping skills that can be deployed in the face of triggers that cannot be avoided. This constitutes the second major component of CBT for addiction, referred to as *coping skills training*. The phrase *recognize–avoid–cope* is commonly used to encompass these broad concepts (Carroll 1998). Essentially, CBT for substance use disorders is an attempt to disrupt the learned association between substance-related cues and use.

Most of what has been written about MI integration has revolved around how it can be incorporated into CBT (Miller and Rollnick 2013). The combination of MI with CBT is intuitive, given the many similarities between them. Specifically, both approaches are collaborative and goal focused, support self-efficacy, and make use of open questions to foster evocation and patient-led problem solving (Flynn 2011). It is important to understand that their differences also contribute to their compatibility and synergistic potential. For example, an important distinction between the two is that MI answers the *why* of behavior change, while CBT informs the *how*. This philosophical subtlety can help one understand why they complement each other so well. Once the patient decides that change is warranted, a slow introduction of CBT concepts can help clarify next steps and thus enhance confidence in the ability to move toward the elaborated goals. This transition must be done in an incremental fashion, because jumping into CBT too quickly can backfire if there is not sufficient motivation to fuel forward momentum. CBT is an active process that does not directly address ambivalence about change, which can represent a missed opportunity to enhance engagement.

Both sequenced and combined approaches can be used to join MI and CBT. As introduced above, a sequenced approach typically involves a slow transition toward CBT once a patient has become fully engaged in the planning phase of MI. For example, when the therapist and the patient are in the process of elaborating a specific change plan, it makes sense to begin shifting gears toward a more CBT-based approach. Other signs that the patient is ready for this shift include the presence of mobilizing change talk, discussion of a clear goal, and the low frequency of sustain talk. Conveniently, there is an organic overlap between the planning stage of MI and the initial session of CBT. Along with the task of introducing the CBT model to the patient, the focus of the first session of CBT for substance use disorders often involves enhancing motivation for change. CBT manuals instruct therapists to do so by eliciting self-motivation statements, listening with empathy, rolling with resistance, clarifying free choice, and looking to identify discrepancies (Carroll 1998). These tasks are highly reminiscent of core MI principles, and this compatibility demonstrates how well CBT dovetails with an MI prelude. Generally speaking, CBT therapists may find MI helpful at treatment outset, as MI is particularly adept at fostering engagement and clarifying goals

Addressing Challenges With Homework Completion

Another practical use of MI within a CBT framework is with the common challenge of homework completion. It has been shown that those who practice CBT skills outside of the therapy hour demonstrate better coping skills and lower substance use (Carroll et al. 2005). Homework noncompletion is commonplace in CBT and can result in frustration on the therapist's part, especially when addressing this issue takes up a majority of session time. CBT therapists often approach this problem by using a cognitive appraisal of the patient's beliefs about doing the homework and rectifying these beliefs as seen fit. If the lack of homework completion is driven by underlying ambivalence about change, the therapist risks falling into the trap of being perceived as authoritatively advocating for change, which may result in the patient arguing for the status quo. An alternative and more collaborative approach would be to recognize and respect the ambivalence, and to use MI skills to help the patient explore and resolve it. The strategies elaborated in Chapter 5 ("Evoking") of this book are particularly useful in this scenario. A vignette is presented below to demonstrate this concept. MI principles are listed in brackets.

> CLINICIAN: John, I sense that it has been difficult in the past few weeks for you to complete our practice exercises outside of session. Is it okay if we take a few minutes to discuss this today? [*Asking for permission*]
> PATIENT: Sure.
> CLINICIAN: First, let me ask you—what are your thoughts about doing the exercises at home? [*Open question*]
> PATIENT: It is just hard for me to find time for it. I have had a lot going on at work lately; things are busy.
> CLINICIAN: It is not possible for you to find time in your schedule for it. [*Amplified reflection*]
> PATIENT: Well I would not say it is impossible, but it would need some planning.
> CLINICIAN: And you have some ideas about how you could make it work...
> [*Complex reflection*]

This approach supports self-efficacy by guiding the patient toward finding his or her own solutions. Once a solution has been identified by the patient, the therapist can then resume the CBT agenda that was put on hold. Another approach that may help in this situation is to invite the patient to choose their homework task among a few possible options, which would emphasize the importance of autonomy. An MI-informed approach can help prevent defensiveness on the patient's part, which often occurs when patients are made to feel like they are not meeting expectations. The techniques described above gently steer the conversation back on course without compromising the therapeutic relationship.

Although the examples above highlight the alternating use of CBT and MI in a complementary fashion, it is also possible to use a combined approach to integrate these two modalities. This allows one to embed MI principles throughout a course of CBT without always needing to switch back and forth between the two.

Enhancing the Therapeutic Alliance

The importance of the therapeutic relationship has been extensively written about, and the quality of the therapeutic relationship consistently stands out as one of the most important active ingredients across psychotherapeutic modalities (Ardito and Rabellino 2011). MI can play an important role in enhancing the quality of the therapeutic relationship. MI is often described as "a way of being" with patients, and the spirit of MI can be maintained throughout the course of other therapies. Its four main components—partnership, acceptance, compassion, and evocation—become the foundation upon which productive therapy can occur.

A helpful example of such a combined approach is the psychotherapy platform used in the COMBINE study, a multicenter study that tested whether combinations of naltrexone, acamprosate, and behavioral interventions would lead to reduced drinking in patients with alcohol dependence (Anton et al. 2006). The behavioral treatment provided in this study—referred to as combined behavioral intervention—consisted of a CBT approach that was delivered according to MI principles. For example, rather than providing an inflexible manualized intervention, the study therapists involved the patient in choosing which modules would be used in his or her own treatment from a menu of different options. This fostering of autonomy and patient-centeredness conjures up the MI spirit, with the goal of enhancing patient engagement. This is important to consider, given that the expert-led culture of CBT can at times clash with MI's premise that the patient holds the answers. Allowing for patient-driven decisions whenever possible while staying within the CBT framework can help mend this discrepancy. A final point worthy of mention is that although we focused on integration of MI with CBT in the context of substance use disorders, the principles described here also apply to CBT for other indications such as mood and anxiety disorders (Arkowitz and Westra 2004).

MOTIVATIONAL INTERVIEWING AND PSYCHODYNAMIC THERAPY

Development of Psychodynamic Theory

Psychodynamic theory has sprouted many branches since its origin as psychoanalysis proper, and its practice has consequently adopted various forms. In general, the term *psychodynamic* is used to refer to any type of therapy that focuses on identifying unconscious psychological phenomena that impact the patient's inner experience or behavior (Gabbard 2014). By gaining insight into these hidden forces, patients acquire the ability to better effect the desired change in their lives (Shedler 2010). Though these general principles are common to all forms of psychodynamic therapy, the existing theories informing how these pathological patterns form and how they can be broken differ substantially.

The psychoanalytic schools of thought borne out of classical Freudian drive theory maintain that human behavior is motivated by sexual and aggressive drives. Freud's tripartite model states that these primitive drives are the domain of the *id*—a purely unconscious phenomenon. *Id* discharge is kept in check by the *ego* and *superego*, which contain both conscious and unconscious elements. Neurotic symptom formation occurs when there is a conflict between these agencies, which leads to the deployment of defense mechanisms (Gabbard 2014). The patient projects his or her unconscious material, which can then be brought to light via interpretations. Taken very literally, the theory implies an "intrapsychic" or one-person model.

Although some of Freud's concepts may be antiquated, part of his creative genius lay in his unabating capacity to revise and develop his theoretical concepts and clinical recommendations. We all are Freudians, and it is inevitable that we claim different parts of Freud's work, which, in turn, we interpret in myriad of ways. It may be that some psychodynamic approaches do not easily lend themselves to integration with MI, whose warmth and connectedness may be at odds with technique rigidity or excessive worry about gratifying transference wishes—though this may not be as problematic as it initially appears to be. We believe that all good therapy is practiced warmly and connectedly, and our choice is not to lock ourselves into any period or variant of Freudian theory, but rather to espouse Freud's spirit of perpetual inquiry, even if it takes us to the later-developed relational psychodynamic approaches.

As psychodynamic scholarship has continued to evolve and branch out, a move toward focusing on the interpersonal realm has emerged. Though the specifics vary among theories, most stipulate that early relationships with caregivers set the frame for one's expectations of others later in life. Non-attuned early relationships lead to psychopathology, as the resulting childhood patterns of beliefs about others persist into adulthood, leading to interpersonal rigidity. For example, a man raised by an unreliable and unavailable parent may grow up to believe that closeness with others is of little use, resulting in an isolated life or a pattern of superficial relationships. In addition to the original focus on the transference cure of psychoanalysis, the extended goal of dynamically based psychotherapy is to provide a *corrective emotional experience* to challenge these expectations and consequently allow the patient's interpersonal repertoire to broaden (Alexander and French 1946). A consistently warm, empathic, and reliable therapist can disprove this patient's maladaptive mental schema. This general framework applies to object relations, self psychology, attachment theory, and interpersonal, relational, and intersubjective relational psychoanalysis (Mitchell and Black 1995). It intuitively follows that the quality of the therapeutic relationship is crucial to the success of therapy. This focus on the interpersonal properties of the therapeutic space overlaps with humanistic psychology, from which MI originated, thus opening the door for integration.

Humanistic psychology originated in the 1950s in response to the yearning for a psychology that focused on human capacity rather than deficits (Schneider et al. 2001). This movement emerged from the Rousseauvian notion that human nature is fundamentally good and that individuals will move toward self-actualization if the right set of conditions is present. From this, it was thought that the study of higher levels of human behavior was the path to understanding the lower or pathological ones. This is in sharp contrast with early psychoanalysis and behaviorism, which sought to understand human behavior by studying those with mental illness and exploring animal models. Carl Rogers is credited with the translation of these principles into the clinical setting, with what he called *person-centered therapy*. In a classic paper, he discussed the essential conditions for the fostering of therapeutic personality change (Rogers 1957). Two of these conditions—namely, *unconditional positive regard* and *accurate empathy*—provided the groundwork for the development of the spirit of MI. Again, the focus on the therapeutic relationship in both MI and relational schools of psychodynamic therapy underlines a compatibility that lends itself well to integration.

Using Motivational Interviewing to Address Substance Use in the Course of Psychodynamic Therapy

MI skills can be powerful when specific behavioral challenges arise in the course of psychodynamic therapy. One common such challenge is substance abuse, which interferes with the consolidation of gained insights and has a negative impact on the individual's ability to participate in the process fully (Dodes 1988). Substance abuse may be the most immediately alarming problem that can be missed or go unaddressed in the course of therapy, and a rigidly applied insight-oriented approach can provoke anxiety and further exacerbate substance use. Our advice here is clear: unless the substance use disorder is approached directly, it is unlikely to improve; and screening for substance use in any therapy gives the opportunity to address the problem by the same provider or to refer to a provider more knowledgeable about addiction treatment. Moreover, it is important to monitor for substance use in the course of any therapy, especially for patients with a history of addiction.

When substance use becomes an issue, it is appropriate to shift gears into an MI style to explore this behavior. Introducing a piece of MI into a psychodynamic core is an example of a sequenced approach to psychotherapy integration. The transition to MI can be done smoothly if an empathic and warm therapeutic stance is adopted from the outset. It can be helpful to signal to the patient when such a switch is being made and to provide the rationale. Highlighting the centrality of experiencing affects to the psychodynamic process, and explaining how substances can hijack this process by artificially manipulating emotional experience, can help in the conversation. This information should not be conveyed in a way that suggests that the patient is "failing" at therapy, but rather it should be framed in a manner that is nonjudgmental and in line with the spirit of MI. Such transparency can enhance engagement and conveys the spirit of collaboration central to MI. The patient vignette below illustrates how this transition can be done. An elicit-provide-elicit approach is employed, as explained in brackets.

> CLINICIAN: I've noticed a change in the process of therapy that I think is worth mentioning. Is it okay if we take a moment to look at this together?" [*Asking for permission*]
> PATIENT: Yeah, sure.
> CLINICIAN: Let me start by asking you if you've noticed anything different as of late? [*Elicit*]
> PATIENT: Well, I know I've missed a few sessions, and I apologize for that. It's been hard to stay focused with the fighting between my husband and me. I've been distracted.
> CLINICIAN: I've certainly gotten that sense too. I would also add that the emotional roller coaster of the past few weeks seems to have resulted in heavier drinking than is typical for you. Do you agree? [*Provide-Elicit*]
> PATIENT: I know, I know. I had been doing well for over a year now, but I'm finding it harder and harder to resist the urge. Sometimes it's the only way I know to shut my brain off.
> CLINICIAN: One of my concerns about this is that the type of therapy we've been doing relies on the ability to sit with emotions, even when these emotions are difficult to bear. A lot of the healing comes from gaining a better understanding of the origin of these difficult feelings, and then learning how to cope with them. Drinking gets in the way of this process [*Provide*]. You've dedicated a lot of time and effort to the work of therapy, and I would hate for your efforts not to be met with good results [*Affirmation*]. What would you think of switching gears for a bit so we can put

our heads together to better understand what's been happening with your
drinking? [*Elicit*]
PATIENT: I guess that makes sense, sure.

Depending on its severity, a brief MI interlude may be sufficient to abort
the lapse to substance use. Alternatively, it may also be necessary to refer the patient for more intensive substance use treatment and to resume psychodynamic
therapy when appropriate. The appropriate timing for switching back to psychodynamic therapy is case specific, and a discussion of this decision is beyond the
scope of this chapter. However, although the *when* will not be discussed here, a
few guidelines about the *how* are examined below.

When the therapist changes to a psychodynamic style after a portion of MI
has been spliced into the treatment, it is important to signal the switch to the patient. One possible way to do so is to ask the patient to reflect on his or her
experience of the change in approach and then use this as an opportunity to
discuss the *here-and-now* of the therapeutic relationship, thus reintroducing psychodynamic technique that incorporates discussion of the dynamics between the
patient and therapist to advance therapeutic goals.

Part of the challenge to this integrated approach lies in the fact that client-
oriented therapy does not stress the concept of transference. Carl Rogers con-
tended that "transference, as a problem, doesn't arise" in client-centered therapy
(Rogers 1951) and explained that the client-centered approach usually acts to
prevent and diffuse transferences by attempting to accept and understand the
patient's attitudes. Surely many would disagree, and we point out that there are
theoretical and practical differences in therapeutic thinking that may pose challenges (as well as opportunities) when the clinician reverts to psychodynamic
therapy after a course of MI. Psychodynamic authors have posited that applying
supportive methods that make the therapist less "invisible," such as advice and
self-disclosure, may pose challenges to analyzing transference when reverting to
insight-oriented psychotherapy (McWilliams 1994; Rockland 2003).

It bears mentioning that applying a psychodynamic framework can be a
powerful aid in helping to understand the underpinnings of the addictive
behavior. A psychological vulnerability common among patients with addictive
disorders is a difficulty tolerating or experiencing affects (Khantzian 2012). The
use of substances to assist in regulating emotions is at the core of Khantzian's
self-medication hypothesis, which postulates that patients use substances to help
deal with negative affective states due to an absence of alternative coping strategies, either secondary to a developmental deficit or as a result of trauma (Khantzian 1997). It follows that much of the work of psychodynamic therapy for
addiction focuses on identifying and exploring affect. The naming of emotions
empowers the individual to manage them in a more conscious and controlled way
so as to lessen their power to trigger relapse (Khantzian 2012). Khantzian's ap-

proach also echoes the principles of MI, in that he advocates for warmth, empathy, and a nonjudgmental curiosity for the patient. This central philosophy overlaps with MI, and the oft-relapsing nature of addictive disorders makes these two therapies dovetail nicely into a complementary treatment. It is important to add that although the self-medication hypothesis is an elegant theory of the psychological reasons for why a person may be prone to start using a substance, or what may hinder adequate treatment if comorbid conditions are left untreated, it does not follow that addiction abates after those initial or ongoing affective states are addressed. Once addiction develops, it becomes a separate disorder that needs to be treated directly. For example, a person may start using a substance to self-medicate depression, but once the person is addicted, merely treating the depression is not expected to result in improvement in the addiction.

A final consideration worthy of mention is that for some patients with addictive disorders, a relapse to substance use during a course of psychodynamic therapy can be a red flag indicating that the therapy is too triggering. Thus, when the therapist is implementing an affect-focused or uncovering psychodynamic technique in patients with a history of substance use disorders, it is important that he or she recognize the powerful potential for relapse in the context of increased anxiety or negative affect, unless the patient has a concrete method for maintaining his or her current pattern without exacerbation. For the subset of patients for whom the increased anxiety of uncovering work is likely to foster an exacerbation of a substance use disorder, a shift toward a more supportive approach is preferable, as described in the next section.

MOTIVATIONAL INTERVIEWING AND SUPPORTIVE PSYCHOTHERAPY

There has been a fair amount of difficulty among psychotherapy writers surrounding the task of defining supportive psychotherapy, especially with respect to its relationship with psychodynamic therapy (Douglas 2008). From a training perspective, the two are taught separately, and the Psychiatry Residency Review Committee consequently lists distinct sets of competencies to be acquired for each modality. A framework has emerged that conceptualizes these two treatment modalities as representing the two ends of a spectrum known as the *supportive-expressive continuum* (Cabaniss et al. 2010). The expressive side of the spectrum represents therapeutic techniques that aim to bring about personality change by fostering the patient's insight into his or her unconscious conflicts. The psychodynamic approaches discussed in the previous section are examples of this style of therapy. On the other hand, the supportive end of the spectrum has the objective of supporting weakened ego functions to engender symptom relief and more adaptive functioning (Cabaniss et al. 2010; Winston et al. 2012). This latter approach is commonly used in the context of medication management visits in psychiatric clinics.

The patient's psychological mindedness and aptitude for reflection on his or her internal experience helps to guide where the therapist situates himself or herself along the supportive-expressive continuum. For example, patients encountered in hospital psychiatry are often not suitable candidates for in-depth exploratory approaches, given the obstacles posed by the high severity of illness and psychiatric comorbidity. This clinical population is more likely to derive benefit from a supportive stance. Another example is that of the aforementioned patient with an addictive disorder who relapses to substance use because of difficulty tolerating the affect or anxiety generated by an expressive mode of therapy. Although these two scenarios call for a therapeutic stance located closer to the supportive side of the spectrum, a skilled therapist will draw on a psychodynamic understanding of the patient to more effectively tailor treatment. Conversely, supportive approaches can be used to reinforce expressive work. An experienced therapist will move back and forth between these two poles as deemed clinically appropriate. This concept echoes the fluidity we advocate for in this chapter with respect to the integration of MI and other psychotherapeutic modalities.

The boundary between supportive psychotherapy and MI is a blurry one. Some have even described MI as a mainstay of supportive treatment for substance use disorder (Winston et al. 2012). Semantics aside, MI can be a great asset in the context of supportive psychotherapy, especially when the issue of behavioral change presents itself. This is especially true when there exists a component of ambivalence. Using a combined approach to integration is most useful in this setting, as MI and supportive psychotherapy merge quite nicely, given the significant overlap in technique and directive strategy (Rosenthal 2008). It is also of note that the four processes of MI—engaging, focusing, evoking, and planning—echo the natural progression of supportive psychotherapy. Thus, MI-specific interventions can easily be drawn on in the context of supportive psychotherapy to help resolve ambivalence and facilitate change, which in turn boosts the potency of the therapy.

Using a Direct, Transparent Communication Style

The most obvious compatibility between supportive psychotherapy and MI is their similar communication style. Supportive psychotherapy texts advocate for a direct, transparent conversational style that strikes a balance between allowing the patient sufficient space to elaborate therapeutically rich material while simultaneously maintaining a reasonable pace (Pinsker 1997; Winston et al. 2012). This approach serves the purpose of reducing anxiety and enhancing the therapeutic relationship. Supportive psychotherapy writers also discourage interrogation-style questioning, which prioritizes acquisition of data at the expense of patient engagement (Pinsker 1997). The MI strategy of following every question with at least two to three reflections provides a useful guide to achieving this balance (Miller and Rollnick 2013). Using a mixture of simple and complex reflections serves to both enhance engagement and promote patient-driven exploration of goals. As in pure MI, the therapist should be mindful to reflect change talk to help guide the patient toward his or her aims.

Yet another point of similarity between MI and supportive psychotherapy is the advice to be mindful of wordiness and speech mannerisms that convey distance (Miller and Rollnick 2013; Pinsker 1997). For example, we can be almost sure that the author of a sentence starting with any of the following lead-in phrases is a therapist: "I'm curious about," "It seems to me," "What I hear you saying." While we all have been heard saying such phrases on occasion, they add little to the flow of the dialogue and might stifle it by conveying detachment rather than warmth and empathy. As Pinsker points out, the routine phrase "I'm curious" suggests that the therapist is concerned with satisfying his or her own curiosity rather than building an alliance with the patient (Pinsker 1997). He adds that a therapist may routinely use such a phrase with patients but will not use it with a superior. Miller and Rollnick (2013) advise therapists to often use the pronoun "you" as the subject of reflections. And so, change talk in this regard can be reflected as "You thought this over and are thinking about using drugs less frequently" rather than "I'm curious about your use of drugs; and from what I hear you saying, it seems to me that you are thinking about using them less frequently."

Facilitating Progress and Dealing With Conflict

In the setting of less structured therapies, such as supportive psychotherapy, it is not uncommon for the beginning therapist to have the impression that the session is "not getting anywhere." This often occurs when a patient has identified the need for behavioral change, but the process of transitioning into action mode is slow to occur. Supportive psychotherapy can often fall prey to this roadblock, and MI can be of help in catalyzing forward momentum. MI accomplishes this task by offering a set of guiding principles that respects the general style of supportive psychotherapy while allowing the therapist to gently guide the process in the direction of positive change. A simple starting strategy consists of employing an abundance of OARS (open questions, affirmations, reflections, and summaries) techniques, as described in previous chapters, with the aim of resolving ambivalence. One can pick and choose among the aforementioned MI techniques, and introduce them into the course of supportive psychotherapy as appropriate.

The "exploring values and goals" approach of MI can be particularly helpful to help a patient move forward when important change decisions need to be made (Miller and Rollnick 2013). This exercise, also known as the *Q technique*, involves having patients sort through cards with a personality characteristic written on each and place them into five piles ranging from "very like me" to "not at all like me." Reading through the cards together provides an opportunity to understand the patients' view of themselves and simultaneously clarifies their values and goals. This can be a powerful tool when the patient and clinician are exploring motivation for a variety of decisions and life changes. Major life events such as career changes, marriage, and divorce often factor into the clinical discourse of supportive psychotherapy. Often, the decision of whether to engage in treatment or not is the one being debated. A common situation in the setting of substance use disorder treatment is ambivalence about engaging in self-help resources such as Alcoholics Anonymous. Using approaches and tools rooted in MI such as the Q technique can be helpful in bringing decisive variables into focus and in promoting further discourse that can eventually encourage patients to make decisions that move them closer to their goals.

Whenever therapy does not proceed as expected, many schools of psychotherapy advise the therapist to consider whether resistance may be at play. *Resistance* can be described as anything the patient does that gets in the way of the therapeutic process (Cabaniss et al. 2011). Although this general definition is widely respected, recommendations on how to respond to it vary broadly. More expressive approaches use resistance as an opportunity for uncovering work that aims to unearth contributing defenses, thus working from the inside out. Supportive approaches generally tackle resistance from the outside in, by attempting to support the person's ability to function and modify the external factors that cause him or her to become "stuck," and only moving toward a more uncovering style when the more directly supportive techniques are insufficient, provided the patient has the capacity and is also willing. Adding MI-informed techniques to the supportive psychotherapy arsenal can greatly help this process along. MI is unique in its reframing resistance as either ambivalence-driven sustain talk or discord in the interpersonal process. It follows from this formulation that further exploration and gradual resolution of ambivalence and mindfully attending to the therapeutic relationship are the two ways to address what might be labeled as "resistance" in other therapeutic modalities. The therapist is encouraged to reflect on where the patient is in the phase of therapy and to ensure that the therapy being delivered matches this stage. For example, a therapist who prematurely jumps into the planning phase of treatment is likely to be met with sustain talk. Similarly, a therapist using a supportive approach should not jump into concrete problem solving and advice giving until the patient is noted to engage in mobilizing change talk. Using an MI lens to remain aware of the patient's perceived readiness for action is essential to ensure that the treatment delivered does not fall wide of the mark.

Enhancing Self-Esteem

The task of enhancing self-esteem is central to supportive psychotherapy, and, unsurprisingly, many pages can be borrowed from the book of MI to achieve this goal (Pinsker 1997). The most obvious strategy consists of being generous with affirmations and taking every opportunity to highlight the patient's strengths and accomplishments. Often this approach represents a shift in the therapist's focus, as most therapists are trained to pick up on deficits rather than strengths. A Rogerian or humanistic approach encourages the opposite—namely, a focus on that which is desirable and adaptive (Rogers 1957).

Another useful MI tool that can serve this function is use of the confidence and importance rulers (Miller and Rollnick 2013; see also Chapter 5, "Evoking," in this book). When discussing a specific behavioral goal, the therapist asks the patient, "On a scale of 0 to 10, with 0 being 'not at all confident' and 10 being 'extremely confident,' how confident are you that you'll be able to make this change?" Once the patient identifies a number, a way to elicit change talk is to ask the patient why he or she chose this number instead of a lower one. This will naturally lead patients to talk about specific reasons why they believe they are able to make the change, simultaneously boosting their confidence. Change talk can be boosted by reflecting it, and the therapist can then apply the same process to address perceived importance by using the importance ruler.

Giving Advice

Though MI and supportive psychotherapy share many similarities, the latter's active and advice-giving style represents a predictable challenge when delivering both therapies jointly. One might initially interpret advice giving as contradictory to the spirit of MI, which states that the answers reside within the patient. However, there are ways in which the therapist may dispense advice while still respecting this principle. Here we discuss two specific strategies for doing so: asking for permission and the elicit-provide-elicit approach. A good rule of thumb when offering advice during the course of supportive psychotherapy is to always ask the patient for permission prior to doing so. This serves to diffuse the therapist-patient power differential that is incongruent with MI. Below is an example of phrasing to ask permission:

> I see that you find yourself in a difficult situation. I know of some things others have found helpful when facing similar problems. Is it okay if I share them with you?

This is not necessary when the patient is the one directly requesting information or advice. Even in this scenario, it is wise to ask the patient what he or she already thinks or knows about the topic prior to offering the information. This not only avoids falling into the trap of "telling the patient what he or she already knows" but also enhances collaboration.

When one dispenses information, the elicit-provide-elicit approach discussed in previous chapters can be instrumental. It is also important to use autonomy-supportive language to emphasize that the patient is in the driver's seat and the therapist is a consultant on the journey. Checking in with the patient after offering information is also good practice, and it promotes identification of disagreements or misunderstandings that may have otherwise been missed.

MOTIVATIONAL INTERVIEWING AND GROUP THERAPY

There are many obvious advantages to providing psychotherapeutic treatment in groups. Not only does this format improve access to treatment in a manner that is cost-effective, but it also allows for tapping into the group's transformative power. Unlike individual therapy, the group setting allows patients more opportunity to recognize and address the interpersonal ramifications of their behavior, creates opportunities to provide and receive valuable feedback, and breaks their isolation by providing living proof that many others struggle with similar difficulties (Yalom and Leszcz 2005).

Although delivery of MI in the group setting has become commonplace in the treatment of substance use disorders, studies have not consistently demonstrated it to be equivalent in efficacy to individual interventions (Miller and Rollnick 2013). One potential explanation for this finding is that behavior change has been found to correlate with the amount of patient change talk per session (Magill et al. 2014). The group format results in reduced airtime per member when compared with individual interventions—an important difference that may lie at the root of the variance in efficacy between individual and group-delivered MI. Despite this, the group format is a reality of our resource-limited treatment settings, and it is therefore worthwhile to discuss ways to enhance MI fidelity in this context.

The general principles of MI—*partnership (collaboration)*, *acceptance*, *compassion*, and *evocation*—apply to the group setting, with the end goal of exploring and resolving ambivalence about change. A critical difference, however, is that the therapist must simultaneously attend to group process—a task that can sometimes pose challenges not encountered in individual treatment. It is essential for the therapist practicing this modality to be proficient in both MI and general group therapy principles, because integrating the two requires a certain degree of sophistication. Beginning therapists who have the luxury of leading groups in pairs may choose to assign a specific role to each group therapist. For example, one may focus on group process while the other focuses on reflections and other OARS skills (Velasquez et al. 2008). Specific considerations for the delivery of MI in the group format are discussed below.

Fostering a Group Culture Consistent With Motivational Interviewing

The establishment of group norms is a crucial early task for all group therapy modalities (Yalom and Leszcz 2005). In the setting of an MI group, introducing the spirit of MI is a prerequisite in the first group meeting. This can be achieved by explicitly describing its philosophy surrounding the process of change, by normalizing ambivalence, and by underlining the importance of autonomy. Here is an example of what such an introduction might sound like:

> Before we get started, I'd like to introduce some of the principles that will help guide how we interact as a group. Everyone in the group is here because there is an aspect of their lives that they are considering changing. Much like we are all unique, and each of us has their own reasons for being here, the solutions are also unique. Because of this, this group discourages giving advice to others, unless they ask for it specifically. Instead, we focus on listening so that together we can better understand what the issues are. This deeper understanding will allow us to help others explore their problems and discover their own solutions. It is also important to mention that change is a process, and people may be at different stages of this process. Some will already have decided that they are ready to make a change. Others will be unsure as to whether they even want to be in this group in the first place. This is normal and expected. It's important to respect everyone's position, and not to pressure them.

These principles may need to be revisited at different points in the course of therapy, or whenever a new member joins if it is an open group. The core message conveyed is that ambivalence is normal and expected, everyone is different, and supporting others by listening and allowing them to come to their own conclusions is what has been found to work best. The therapist will demonstrate these group norms by way of example and by modeling core MI-consistent behaviors such as OARS skills. Group members will look to the therapist for guidance and typically will follow suit, especially once they witness how this open and empathic approach is often successful at eliciting change talk.

Responding to Group Behavior That Is Inconsistent With Motivational Interviewing

Despite best efforts to introduce the group to the climate of MI, there will be times when group members do not adhere to these principles. It then becomes the therapist's role to address this departure from group norms. A common MI-inconsistent behavior is excessive focus on "solution talk," which is often a learned behavior from more skills-based group therapies. These advice-giving interludes usually stem from a desire to help, and this underlying motivation should be mentioned by the therapist in order to prevent their intervention from sounding critical. A "reframe-remind-return" framework has been elaborated to help maneuver around this issue, and the following example shows how a therapist might intervene when a group member offers unsolicited advice to another member (Krejci and Neugebauer 2015).

> James, I can see that you want to share your own experience to help Emma with her current difficulties, and it's clear that you want to help. Let me just interject

here that in this type of group, we try to stay away from giving advice, unless directly asked for it. Emma, you've been going through a rough time as of late. How were you hoping the group could support you today?

The therapist ought not be hesitant to jump in when such a scenario occurs. Similar interjections may be necessary when group members are critical of one another. Reminding members of the importance of a nonjudgmental stance and an attitude of positive curiosity can be helpful. Standard group therapy interventions designed to maintain respect can be used, such as the encouragement of "I" statements, which tend to reduce the critical punch of pointed remarks. Asking the receiver of criticism to openly express how the comment was experienced may provide a helpful here-and-now intervention to promote cohesion and interpersonal learning. The spirit of MI is the catalyst that allows the process of change to unfold, and it should be promoted and protected judiciously.

Balancing Individual and Group Interventions

One of the challenges of delivering MI in a group format is that one must prevent the sessions from becoming a series of short segments of individualized interventions. This siloed approach risks losing other group members' engagement, especially if discussions are too narrowly tailored to the group member being addressed. A helpful strategy includes the use of *reflective statements* and *summaries* to amplify general themes, rather than the specifics of an individual's situation. For example, instead of focusing on a particular conversation between a group member and his spouse who berated him for not quitting smoking, the group leader can choose to focus on the experience of being pressured into things one is ambivalent about. Of course, while doing this the group leader should strive to selectively reflect change talk and always be on the lookout for opportunities to provide *affirmations*. Here is an example:

> David, you're continuing to experience a lot of pressure from your family to quit smoking; but despite the frustration this triggers, you've managed to stick to your plan to reduce how much you smoke, and you've continued to come to this group! Sara, this reminds me of when you felt belittled by your doctor when he criticized you for your drinking and, like David, you didn't let that steer you off course. Has anyone else in the group had similar experiences?

Recruiting group members to share their own related experiences is validating and simultaneously engaging.

Another helpful strategy is to invite other members to weigh in when a general topic is brought up. Once a few group members have spoken about a general topic, the therapist can then use a *summary statement* to unite the various contributions. Meeting with prospective group members for individual assessments prior to them joining the group can be quite helpful with this approach, because it affords the group leader strategic knowledge about which topics are likely to be universally germane.

Some of the standard MI tools may be adapted to the group format fairly seamlessly and may be used to simultaneously engage many members. One such example is the use of the "ruler technique." A confidence (or importance) ruler with markings from 0 to 10 can be drawn on the board (see Figures 5–2 and 5–3 in Chapter 5), and individual members are then invited to write their names on the ruler where they would rate their confidence in their ability to make the proposed change. The ruler can then be used as in individual therapy—with each member taking turns to explain why they did not choose a lower number and subsequently what it would take for the number to increase, so as to elicit change talk. As in individual MI, change talk can then be reflected. There are many such ways to creatively make use of the group to promote engagement. It is crucial, however, to be mindful of the important task of maximizing the amount of *mobilizing change talk* for each individual, because this is the ingredient most strongly associated with change (Magill et al. 2014).

KEY POINTS

- Motivational interviewing (MI) can be woven into other psychotherapy modalities using either a *sequenced* or a *combined* approach.

- *Sequenced* approaches consist of using two or more psychotherapy techniques in an alternating manner. These approaches are most useful when the clinician is addressing low motivation in the context of a psychotherapeutic modality other than MI. Examples include

  - Using an MI prelude prior to starting cognitive-behavioral therapy (CBT) to enhance motivation and to establish a strong therapeutic alliance.

  - Inserting a piece of MI to address homework noncompliance during CBT.

  - Using an MI-informed approach to address relapse to substance use during the course of psychodynamic therapy (or other modalities).

- *Combined* approaches to integration blend elements of MI within the framework of a second form of psychotherapy to form a synergistic whole. Examples include

  - Using OARS (open questions, affirmations, reflections, summaries) skills to enhance forward momentum in the context of supportive psychotherapy that targets behavioral change.

- Using open-ended questions and reflective statements to explore ambivalence about pursuing treatment modalities and resources (e.g., pharmacotherapy, Alcoholics Anonymous attendance).

- Using affirmations to enhance self-esteem, which is a core goal of supportive psychotherapy.

- Asking for permission or using the elicit-provide-elicit approach to promote a sense of collaboration when giving advice in the context of supportive psychotherapy.

- MI can be delivered in a group format. Important tasks to consider when doing so include

  - Educating group members about the spirit of MI.

  - Intervening promptly when MI-inconsistent behaviors occur.

  - Balancing group and individual interventions.

  - Maximizing change talk.

STUDY QUESTIONS

1. Which of the following psychotherapy integration approaches was Carl Rogers a proponent of?

   A. Theoretical integration.
   B. Common factors.
   C. Assimilative integration.
   D. Additive combining.
   E. Technical eclecticism.

2. The first session of cognitive-behavioral therapy (CBT) for substance use disorders overlaps most with which motivational interviewing (MI) process?

   A. Engaging.
   B. Focusing.
   C. Evoking.
   D. Planning.
   E. Concluding.

3. The spirit of MI is most consistent with which of the following?

    A. Freudian drive theory.
    B. Object relations theory.
    C. Humanistic psychology.
    D. Self psychology.
    E. Attachment theory.

4. Which of the following MI techniques is most helpful for giving advice to patients during a course of supportive psychotherapy?

    A. Reframe-remind-return.
    B. Complex reflective statements.
    C. Amplified reflections.
    D. Inform-reframe-inform.
    E. Elicit-provide-elicit.

5. Which of the following statements is *true* regarding MI delivered in a group setting?

    A. The therapist should use reflections to amplify "solution talk" by group members.
    B. MI delivered in groups is as efficacious as individually delivered MI.
    C. Group members should all be in the same "stage of change."
    D. Therapists should strive to maximize mobilizing change talk for each group member.
    E. Each group session should focus on one to two group members.

REFERENCES

Alexander F, French TM: Psychoanalytic Therapy: Principles and Application. New York, Ronald Press, 1946, p 66

Anton RF, O'Malley SS, Ciraulo DA, et al: Combined pharmacotherapies and behavioral interventions for alcohol dependence: the COMBINE study: a randomized controlled trial. JAMA 295(17):2003–2017, 2006 16670409

Ardito RB, Rabellino D: Therapeutic alliance and outcome of psychotherapy: historical excursus, measurements, and prospects for research. Front Psychol 2:270, 2011 22028698

Arkowitz H, Westra HA: Integrating motivational interviewing and cognitive behavioral therapy in the treatment of depression and anxiety. J Cogn Psychother 18(4):337–350, 2004

Brady KT, Dansky BS, Back SE, et al: Exposure therapy in the treatment of PTSD among cocaine-dependent individuals: preliminary findings. J Subst Abuse Treat 21(1):47–54, 2001 11516926

Cabaniss DL, Arbuckle MR, Douglas C: Beyond the supportive-expressive continuum: an integrated approach to psychodynamic psychotherapy in clinical practice. Focus 8(1):25–31, 2010

Cabaniss DL, Cherry S, Douglas CJ, et al: Psychodynamic Psychotherapy. New York, Wiley, 2011

Carroll KM: A Cognitive-Behavioral Approach: Treating Cocaine Addiction. Therapy Manuals for Drug Abuse, Manual 1. NIH Publ No 98-4308. Rockville, MD, National Institute on Drug Abuse, April 1998

Carroll KM, Onken LS: Behavioral therapies for drug abuse. Am J Psychiatry 162(8):1452–1460, 2005 16055766

Carroll KM, Nich C, Ball SA: Practice makes progress? Homework assignments and outcome in treatment of cocaine dependence. J Consult Clin Psychol 73(4):749–755, 2005 16173864

Dodes LM: The psychology of combining dynamic psychotherapy and Alcoholics Anonymous. Bull Menninger Clin 52(4):283–293, 1988 3042066

Douglas CJ: Teaching supportive psychotherapy to psychiatric residents. Am J Psychiatry 165(4):445–452, 2008 18381914

Flynn HA: Setting the stage for the integration of motivational interviewing with cognitive behavioral therapy in the treatment of depression. Cognit Behav Pract 18(1):46–54, 2011

Gabbard GO: Psychodynamic Psychiatry in Clinical Practice, 5th Edition. Washington, DC, American Psychiatric Publishing, 2014

Hettema J, Steele J, Miller WR: Motivational interviewing. Annu Rev Clin Psychol 1:91–111, 2005 17716083

Khantzian EJ: The self-medication hypothesis of substance use disorders: a reconsideration and recent applications. Harv Rev Psychiatry 4(5):231–244, 1997 9385000

Khantzian EJ: Reflections on treating addictive disorders: a psychodynamic perspective. Am J Addict 21(3):274–279, discussion 279, 2012 22494231

Krejci J, Neugebauer Q: Motivational interviewing in groups: group process considerations. Journal of Groups in Addiction & Recovery 10(1):23–40, 2015

Magill M, Gaume J, Apodaca TR, et al: The technical hypothesis of motivational interviewing: a meta-analysis of MI's key causal model. J Consult Clin Psychol 82(6):973–983, 2014 24841862

McWilliams N: Psychoanalytic Dagnosis. New York, Guilford, 1994

Miller WR, Rollnick S: Motivational Interviewing: Helping People Change, 3rd Edition. New York, Guilford, 2013

Mitchell SA, Black MJ: Freud and Beyond: A History of Modern Psychoanalytic Thought. New York, Basic Books, 1995

Najavits LM, Weiss RD: The role of psychotherapy in the treatment of substance-use disorders. Harv Rev Psychiatry 2(2):84–96, 1994 9384886

Pinsker H: A Primer of Supportive Psychotherapy. Hillsdale, NJ, Analytic Press, 1997

Rockland LH: Supportive Therapy. New York, Basic Books, 2003

Rogers CR: Client-Centered Therapy: Its Current Practice, Implications and Theory. London, Constable, 1951

Rogers CR: The necessary and sufficient conditions of therapeutic personality change. J Consult Psychol 21(2):95–103, 1957 13416422

Rosenthal RN: Techniques of individual supportive psychotherapy, in Textbook of Psychotherapeutic Treatments. Edited by Gabbard GO. Washington, DC, American Psychiatric Publishing, 2008, pp 417–445

Schneider KJ, Bugental JFT, Pierson JF: The Handbook of Humanistic Psychology. Thousand Oaks, CA, Sage, 2001

Shedler J: The efficacy of psychodynamic psychotherapy. Am Psychol 65(2):98–109, 2010 20141265

Stricker G, Gold J: Psychotherapy integration: an assimilative psychodynamic approach. Clin Psychol Sci Pract 3:47–58, 1996

Velasquez MM, Stephens NS, Ingersoll K: Motivational interviewing in groups. Journal of Groups in Addiction & Recovery 1:27–50, 2008

Winston A, Rosenthal RN, Pinsker H: Learning Supportive Psychotherapy: An Illustrated Guide. Washington, DC, American Psychiatric Publishing, 2012

Yalom ID, Leszcz M: The Theory and Practice of Group Psychotherapy, 5th Edition. New York, Basic Books, 2005

STUDENT REFLECTIONS

Augustine Tawadros

Rutgers New Jersey Medical School, MS-III

As new forms of psychotherapy arise, it's important to reflect on whether they can be compatible with each other and enhance the way treatments are implemented. This chapter demonstrates how well motivational interviewing (MI) complements other psychotherapeutic approaches and how one can customize a treatment plan tailored to a patient's needs. It is critical to acknowledge, as highlighted in the chapter, that a rigid treatment plan is detrimental to the patient and that instead therapeutic flexibility should be the approach taken.

It is helpful to take integrated therapeutic approaches and also use them as guidelines when treating patients medically. As physicians, it's important to establish a good rapport with patients, since it will boost and enhance a goal-focused treatment plan. For example, in the chapter, the authors explain that using MI skills with cognitive-behavioral therapy in exploring why patients have a hard time completing exercises at home can help patients find their own answers. The same technique can be applied in allowing patients to search for solutions as to why they are not complying with doctor's orders. For instance, a physician may give instructions about dietary restrictions to a patient but at the same time should encourage active patient participation in the treatment plan to give the patient a sense of ownership and responsibility. This is especially important when trying to combine strategies in order to enrich a successful plan.

After you read this chapter on MI, it's critical to remember that a patient's needs will change significantly throughout the treatment process and a doctor must have the knowledge and the skill to adapt and adjust the plan to meet the patient's goals. The main theme of the chapter is to show how MI can be combined with other therapies to create a more distinct treatment plan for each patient. This emphasis has enlightened my mindset in medicine and has showed me that there is no strict solution but, rather, that different approaches should be integrated and analyzed together in order to maximize recovery.

Motivational Interviewing and Pharmacotherapy

SueAnn Kim, M.D.
Vicki Kalira, M.D.

> When someone really hears you without passing judgment on you, without trying to take responsibility for you, without trying to mold you, it feels damn good.
>
> —*Carl Rogers*

> True life is lived when tiny changes occur.
>
> —*Leo Tolstoy*

The standard of care for behavioral change in most patients involves a combination of medication and psychosocial interventions. For acute conditions, providers typically ask symptom-specific questions and prescribe short-term medication accordingly. Conversely, the management of chronic illness requires sustained behavioral change; therefore, a supportive, empathic, and collaborative approach is employed. In addition, a strong therapeutic alliance, effective communication, and continued motivation have a significant impact on adherence to medications.

In the first part of this chapter, we demonstrate how the principles of motivational interviewing (MI) can be utilized throughout the shared decision-making process about medications by building the foundation of a respectful patient-provider relationship, resolving ambivalence, supporting patient actions, and addressing adherence. In the second part, we review U.S. Food and Drug Administration (FDA)–approved medications for the treatment of substance use disorders. In doing so, we consider how motivational work can impact the choice of the medication from the perspective of the provider and the patient. Finally, we consider the application of these principles in a clinical example.

MOTIVATIONAL INTERVIEWING PRINCIPLES AND MEDICATIONS

Engaging

Irrespective of which treatment model one employs, a strong therapeutic relationship is central to fostering a patient's engagement and participation in treatment. Patients who trust their providers demonstrate improved adherence; they are also more satisfied and comfortable with their care, communicate better, and are more likely to disclose information (Martin et al. 2005). Additionally, these patients remain in treatment longer, which correlates with improved outcomes. Therefore, the strength and quality of the alliance is considered at least as important as the intervention being offered. Providers may wish to consider the following strategies in order to better engage patients in pharmacological management.

Avoid the Assessment Trap

During the initial interview, it is tempting to use a series of directed questions common in structured evaluations in the interest of time and in an effort to focus the session. However, this narrows the conversation by putting the provider's objectives into focus, rather than the patient's needs and goals. It also puts patients in a passive role, rather than the active, engaged role needed for eventual success.

Allow Patients to Be Heard

Rather than launching into a barrage of questions, asking open questions permits more time for listening in lieu of talking. Even in a fast-paced clinic, the value of allowing patients to express themselves uninterrupted does not have to come at the expense of additional time. By using the MI skills of asking open questions, affirming, reflecting, and summarizing (OARS), providers simultaneously show respect and express empathy, concern, and understanding. Patients subsequently perceive this experience as being more important than the actual amount of time spent with the provider (Dorr Goold and Lipkin 1999). To ensure that all the necessary questions have been addressed, the provider may discuss with the patient the fact that a portion of the session will be reserved for asking specific questions in contrast to the initial open-ended format.

Resist the Righting Reflex

While the provider may have a pharmacological approach in mind, he or she should resist falling into the expert role of immediately offering this advice (the so-called righting reflex). Even in situations where the use of medications seems inherent (e.g., in a methadone clinic), patients may not be ready to commit despite coming to the appointment. Offering or even defending the need for medications without attending to the patient's concerns can unwittingly disengage the patient and foster mistrust. It may also suggest a lack of appreciation for the complex issues that surround the decision to take medications.

Buber eloquently said, "I have not the right to want to change another if I am not open to be changed by him" (Anderson and Cissna 1997, p. 21). While providers may be experts in pharmacotherapy, patients are experts on themselves, and we should utilize their expertise. The patient is the one who will choose whether or not to engage in and adhere to treatment. The patient is the one who will provide information as to how the treatment is progressing. The patient knows what has worked in the past and what may be most helpful in their current situation. The shared decision making that follows is consistent with the spirit of MI.

Focusing

After the initial assessment, the provider and the patient collaboratively establish the focus of treatment. Often the patient may have one objective in mind and the provider another. Medications themselves may not be the initial focus of the patient, but the patient may have other behavior changes he or she wants to work on. Additionally, certain medications may not be suitable at a given time if they are inconsistent with the goals of the patient. For example, if a patient's aim is not abstinence from alcohol, disulfiram is not a great option. Note that focusing should still incorporate the provider's recommendations, based on evidence, in an interactive exchange of information with the patient.

Exchanging Information

Oftentimes patients may not be aware of the role of medication in substance use treatment. An important role of the provider is to share valuable information about pharmacotherapy and provide evidence-based recommendations. The skillful presentation of such knowledge based on MI principles helps to increase a patient's receptiveness to potentially life-saving information about pharmacotherapy. Using the MI strategy of elicit-provide-elicit engages patients in an exchange that builds on their personal knowledge and experience, assesses their understanding of newly presented information, and allows for feedback. It avoids a paternalistic and overbearing approach that risks disengaging the patient from treatment. Providers may want to

Elicit:

- Ask what the patient already knows about medications: "What do you know about medications for alcohol addiction?"

- Ask permission to share information: "Is it okay to share some information about medications that others have found useful?"

Provide:

- Use easy-to-understand concepts and basic language: "Medication can help a person stop thinking about drugs all the time."
- Use a menu of options when possible: "There are different types of treatment settings that offer different types of medications."
- Deliver information in the context of other patients: "Patients in similar situations as yourself have been maintained on medications safely for years."
- Provide written information for subsequent review and to share with loved ones.

Elicit:

- Ask what the patient thinks: "What are your thoughts?"

Accepting the Patient

Acknowledging a patient's right to make an informed decision not only helps the patient open up to recommendations but also preserves the therapeutic alliance should the patient disagree with treatment options. Therefore, providers can continue to address possible concerns, questions, stigma, and misconceptions, as well as develop alternative strategies over time. Providers may wish to spend more time further engaging the patient in a dialogue by building rapport, exploring values, and affirming strengths.

Evoking

Once a change goal is identified through focusing, the provider can then evoke the patient's own motivations or plans for change. If the use of medications is consistent with one's goals, remember that MI does not exempt the need for informed consent. Once informed consent is obtained, the provider should listen for change talk and evoke confidence: "You want to try buprenorphine to help with your pain and feelings of being out of control, but you are afraid you won't be able to do it. How were you able to do it before?" The provider may even preemptively acknowledge that taking medications is difficult, in order to facilitate an open discussion about the patient's concerns (Willey 1999). Expressing empathy and understanding allows the patient to feel comfortable to discuss doubts and provides opportunities to identify change talk and reflect confidence statements; however, the provider may need to take a step back and explore alternate perspectives and strategies, including stopping the medication. In an MI-consistent way, the provider can offer a counterbalance to the patient's focus on the negative aspects of taking medications through open questions and reflections that increase attention on the potential benefits, and actively work toward increasing change talk. This is done by utilizing the patient's own statements supporting behavioral change and evoking the patient's own desire, ability, reasons, and need for change.

Once there has been adequate dialogue to ensure that the patient has the information he or she needs to provide informed consent, the provider can discuss the patient's ambivalence about utilizing medication-assisted treatment. *Ambivalence* reflects conflicting but co-occurring attitudes that typically stall action. Despite advantages to taking medications such as reduced cravings or symptoms, there are disadvantages such as stigma, side effects, dietary restrictions, laboratory monitoring, or frequent clinic visits. Also, patients may not feel confident in their ability to overcome monetary, logistical, societal, or psychological barriers required to take medications. Providers may feel frustrated when patients leave prescriptions unfilled, take doses irregularly, or abruptly discontinue medication. They may perceive patients as being "resistant" or "noncompliant." Yet, ambivalence is a normal part of change, and in the evoking process of MI, providers can work with patients to address their ambivalence toward taking medications and enhance adherence with additional strategies.

Increasing Change Talk

Providers can listen carefully for change talk that favors taking medications and reinforce such statements using key MI communication skills: open questions, affirmation, reflections, or summaries. Providers may also evoke change talk by engaging patients in discussions about their desire, ability, reasons, or need to treat their substance use and willingness to take medications as a part of their recovery.

Building Self-Efficacy

As Bandura (1977) noted, "Efficacy expectations determine how much effort people will expend and how long they will persist in the face of obstacles and aversive experiences" (p. 194). When patients believe they can succeed in a behavioral change, they are more likely to initiate and sustain that change. In fact, high self-efficacy has been shown to correlate with greater medication adherence (Krueger et al. 2005). Therefore, evoking confidence talk by affirming a patient's strengths or reviewing past accomplishments in treatment is a key component of using MI to increase self-efficacy.

Planning

During the evoking process, patients may have committed to taking medications without considering or understanding what that entails. It is difficult to take medication every single day. In addition, not planning on ways to manage cravings or relapse can be dangerous, especially in the case of certain medications like disulfiram (discussed later in this chapter). In an MI-consistent manner, the provider and patient can create an individualized plan. The provider can offer a menu of options, while asking permission to share clinically relevant information and ultimately focus the plan back on the patient's expressed goals.

Following Up

While it may seem as if the goal has been achieved and the job complete once the patient is engaged in the behavioral change that he or she committed to and planned for, the plan may have to be modified. During the initial or subsequent visits, the provider can elicit ways in which previous obstacles have been overcome or offer information as to what has been helpful for others in similar situations. It's natural for the patient to revert to ambivalence in the setting of difficulty. The provider may find it helpful to continue engaging the patient, enhancing self-efficacy, affirming the patient's efforts and accomplishments, focusing on specific goals or concerns, eliciting change talk, and allowing for new specific, patient-generated plans.

Sustaining Adherence

One of the common goals for effective treatment is sustained medication adherence. This can be particularly challenging, because it requires ongoing commitment from the patient and the provider to the plan and each other. Throughout medicine, adherence to medication for chronic diseases ranges widely, with an average of 50% (Nieuwlaat et al. 2014), while adherence rates are lower for patients with substance use as well as psychiatric illness (Magura et al. 2014).

Most often, the provider is unaware that a patient is struggling with an established treatment plan. The patient may not spontaneously volunteer his or her difficulties with taking medications. This can be the result of misunderstanding, shame, fear, or a desire to please the provider. An opportunity to intervene may be missed if the provider does not directly ask about adherence to medications, and the patient may not truthfully respond if the questioning is done in a judgmental or MI-inconsistent manner. Offering information and advising the patient that nonadherence is not a valuation of his or her character as "good" or "bad" encourages the patient to speak openly. The spirit of partnership in MI provides a base to work with the patient to come up with solutions.

MEDICATIONS FOR SUBSTANCE USE DISORDERS

Medications aid motivational, behavioral, and other psychosocial interventions for substance use treatment by targeting withdrawal symptoms and physiological cravings and by mitigating euphoric effects. Despite evidence of improved clinical outcomes, medications remain underutilized (Mark et al. 2009; Roman et al. 2011). One barrier to physician prescribing may be physicians' own lack of knowledge, perception of effectiveness, concern about side effects, and lack of time to prescribe or follow up (Mark et al. 2003). In an effort to address this potential barrier, we offer the following overview of medications commonly used in relapse prevention and suggestions on how to integrate MI with specific medications, as a starting point for prescribers to consider if integrating this strategy into their practice (Table 8–1).

Alcohol Use Disorder

People who struggle with alcohol use disorder represent a cohort with various therapeutic goals and needs. Decision making among this heterogeneous group should balance the patient's preferences alongside one's own clinical judgment (Center for Substance Abuse Treatment 2009). The medications in Table 8–2 differ in mechanism of action, administration, adverse events, and availability.

Disulfiram

Given the severity of the disulfiram-ethanol reaction, patients must receive careful counseling with abstinence as the goal. Although outcomes on duration of abstinence and days of heavy drinking are better with other medications (Jonas et al. 2014), disulfiram provides a physical deterrent to alcohol use that may be appropriate for patients who waver in their motivation to remain abstinent at specific times (e.g., holidays, birthdays). While this external motivation may help achieve sobriety, it is important to explore whether the patient views his or her sobriety purely as a mechanism of the medication, because this may impede the strengthening of self-motivation and self-efficacy, which are crucial to build on to maintain long-term change (Center for Substance Abuse Treatment 1999).

As discussed above, sustained adherence may be difficult with disulfiram, as some patients may stop it in the setting of a planned relapse. However, the provider may be blinded to this if he or she does not ask the patient about adherence in the first place. Once engaged in a dialogue with the patient, the provider may discover new ambivalence or find out that the patient has had a recent relapse. The next step would be to return to focusing on the patient's treatment goals, because they may have changed. The provider may need to switch medications or stop them altogether. If the patient desires to continue with treatment using disulfiram, the provider should consider facilitating supervised administration with the patient's approval.

Naltrexone

Naltrexone is particularly effective in patients with high alcohol cravings and in those whose goal is to reduce heavy drinking (Center for Substance Abuse Treatment 2009). Effectiveness of naltrexone is greatest with consistent use, but rates of adherence tend to be lower among patients who engage in heavy drinking (Kranzler et al. 2003). Therefore, preemptively discussing medication adherence in the evoking stage will likely improve overall effectiveness. Much as

TABLE 8–1. Motivational interviewing and medications by substance use disorder

Alcohol use disorder	Opioid use disorder	Nicotine use disorder
Disulfiram when abstinence is the goal.	Methadone for maintenance. Daily administration in a clinic.	Nicotine replacement alone when motivation is high. Alternatively, consider combination therapy.
Naltrexone when abstinence or reduction in drinking is the goal.	Buprenorphine for maintenance. May be prescribed monthly, office based.	Bupropion SR for facilitating a shift into action. Consider in comorbid depression.
Acamprosate when abstinence or reduction in drinking is the goal. Requires motivation to adhere to three-times-a-day dosing.	Extended-release naltrexone for those patients who cannot take an agonist. There are insufficient Centers for Disease Control and Prevention data to recommend oral formulation.	Varenicline for facilitating a shift into action, especially for those patients without comorbid depression.

TABLE 8–2. Medications for alcohol use disorder

Agent	FDA approval	Mechanism of action	Common side effects	Relative contraindications	Typical dosage and labs; comments
Disulfiram	1951	Inhibits aldehyde dehydrogenase	Headache Fatigue	Any ethanol use Psychosis Severe cardiac disease Severe liver disease Pregnancy	250 mg/day Liver function No ethanol for 12 hours prior to initiation
Naltrexone	1994	μ Opioid receptor antagonist	Nausea Dizziness	Opioid use Liver failure or acute hepatitis	50 mg/day Liver function
Extended-release naltrexone	2006	μ Opioid receptor antagonist	Nausea Headache Injection site pain	Opioid use Liver failure or acute hepatitis	380 mg/4 weeks Liver function
Acamprosate	2004	Unclear, thought to modulate GABA and glutamate	Diarrhea Headache	Renal impairment	666 mg TID Renal function

Note. This table is a summary only and is not meant to reflect a comprehensive review of the medications listed. FDA=U.S. Food and Drug Administration; GABA=γ-aminobutyric acid.

with disulfiram, some patients prefer to use naltrexone in anticipation of high-risk situations, as opposed to daily. When discussing different treatment options in the focusing stage, patients who prefer an alternative to taking a pill every day may be better suited for injectable naltrexone.

Although it is impossible to predict outcomes with any particular patient, it now appears that a certain genetic subgroup of patients responds better to naltrexone: those with a family history of alcoholism, those with early-onset drinking problems, and those who experience a "high" with alcohol (Center for Substance Abuse Treatment 2009). Providers are encouraged to discuss the use of naltrexone specifically in this population.

Acamprosate

Acamprosate appears to reduce subclinical withdrawal symptoms, such as insomnia, anxiety, and restlessness, and helps mitigate cravings and negative reinforcement associated with relapse (Center for Substance Abuse Treatment 2009). The benefits of acamprosate include minimal side effects and drug-drug interactions, as well as safe use in liver disease (Center for Substance Abuse Treatment 2009). However, the patient must remember to take the medication three times a day, and this required regimen needs to be discussed in planning. Providers are encouraged to regularly gauge the level of adherence and strategize with the patient on ways to improve it, such as by using phone reminders or enlisting family support, if the patient remains motivated to use acamprosate.

Opioid Use Disorder

Medication-Assisted Treatment

Medication-assisted treatment (MAT) is the standard of care in opioid use disorder (Table 8–3). It significantly reduces the need for inpatient detoxification, increases treatment retention, improves quality of life, and lowers the risk of exposure to diseases such as hepatitis C and HIV. MAT also reduces illicit opioid use and the risk of fatal overdose. Despite benefits, utilization remains low: only 28% of treatment plans for primary heroin users incorporate MAT (Substance Abuse and Mental Health Services Administration, Center for Behavioral Health Statistics and Quality 2012).

Opioid Replacement Therapy

Opioid replacement therapy comprises methadone and buprenorphine. Methadone is a full μ opioid agonist and buprenorphine is a μ opioid partial agonist. Of note, methadone can only be distributed through specialty opioid treatment programs if the indication is for an opioid use disorder. Although methadone treatment facilities can provide comprehensive counseling and psychiatric services, the restraints of presenting for daily dosing may be a barrier. Conversely, buprenorphine can be prescribed as an office-based treatment. To deter intra-

TABLE 8–3. Medications for opioid use disorder

Agent	FDA approval	Mechanism of action	Common side effects	Relative contraindications	Typical dosage and labs; comments
Methadone	1972	μ Opioid agonist	Drowsiness Constipation Dose-related prolonged QTc	Not part of clinic Severe cardiac disease Severe liver disease Use of alcohol and sedatives (because of interaction)	≥60 mg/day Liver function, ECG
Buprenorphine (often used with naloxone)	2002	μ Opioid partial agonist	Drowsiness Constipation Nausea	Use of other opioids Pregnancy (in which case buprenorphine is used without naloxone) Use of alcohol and sedatives?	16–24 mg/day Liver function, ECG
Extended-release injectable naltrexone	2010	μ Opioid receptor antagonist	Nausea Headache Injection site pain	Opioid use Liver failure or acute hepatitis	380 mg/month Liver function

Note.   This table is a summary only and is not meant to reflect a comprehensive review of the medications listed. ECG=electrocardiogram.

venous misuse, buprenorphine is typically used in a formulation with naloxone (see subsection "Naloxone" later in this section).

Extended-Release Injectable Naltrexone

Agonist treatment with methadone or buprenorphine has the best treatment outcomes (Connery 2015); however, extended-release injectable naltrexone is an alternative when agonists are not an option or not preferred by the patient. This option may be considered more so in patients with concurrent alcohol use disorder, as it might serve a dual purpose (Center for Substance Abuse Treatment 2009). Although it is highly effective at blocking opioid effects, oral naltrexone typically has very poor patient adherence, similar to that with disulfiram (Connery 2015), and is not usually recommended in opioid use disorders.

Medication-Assisted Treatment Versus Detoxification

Talking to patients about opioid use disorder treatment presents unique challenges. While the standard of care is MAT with methadone or buprenorphine, it is not unusual for some patients to prefer detoxification alone. Given the high relapse rates and mortality associated with detoxification without MAT, we encourage providers to strongly recommend maintenance treatment with buprenorphine or methadone as the safest treatment options and extended-release injectable naltrexone as an alternative. Providers should recommend against detoxification alone in patients with an opioid use disorder. Oral naltrexone presents challenges similar those with disulfiram, but unlike disulfiram it has not been shown to be effective. Such a direct message may not seem in line with MI, but recall that it's the provider's responsibility to relay recommendations based on evidenced-based medicine. As always, this dialogue is best done with the patient's permission, so that "the expert trap" can be avoided and a therapeutic collaboration can be maintained. Some patients may remain steadfast in their decision to pursue detoxification over maintenance; however, having a strong therapeutic alliance and respecting patients' autonomy provides ongoing opportunities to discuss MAT if indicated and agreed on in the future.

Naloxone

Naloxone reverses the effects of opioids. It is used as emergency treatment of known or suspected opioid overdose. With the rise in opioid-related deaths in the United States, increasing naloxone distribution to individuals in the community became an important national public health issue. Naloxone can be administered intramuscularly, subcutaneously, intranasally, or via auto-injector. The onset of action is about 2–3 minutes and lasts about 30–90 minutes, after which another dose of naloxone may be needed. When counseling patients on the use of naloxone, it is imperative to explain that administration should always be done in conjunction with calling for emergency medical services because the effects of naloxone are short-lived.

A provider should make it a point to ask permission to provide all patients and their loved ones with information about naloxone, given its ability to save lives. Patients themselves may have heard about it already and ask for points of clarification, and providers can consider starting by asking them what their understanding is first and build on that foundation. Alternatively, the following can be considered to initiate a dialogue: "Can I talk to you about a life-saving medication called naloxone?"

Tobacco Use Disorder

Tobacco use disorder causes devastating health consequences and, according to the Centers for Disease Control and Prevention (2015), is the leading cause of preventable death in the United States. Available pharmacotherapies have proven to be effective in smoking cessation and are considered first-line treatment (Table 8–4).

Patients who are interested in quitting can be offered a menu of options. Bupropion SR or varenicline may minimize ambivalence about quitting if this medication is started prior to the quit date. Nicotine replacement therapy (NRT) is the most widely accessible medication for managing the withdrawal symptoms, cravings, and reinforcing effects of nicotine (Talwar et al. 2004). NRTs can be combined with one another and also with bupropion or varenicline. Bupropion can also be combined with varenicline or NRT. Despite the fact that NRTs increase quit rates by 50%–70% (Stead et al. 2012), the patient may remain ambivalent or prefer to avoid medications altogether. As with MAT, the provider should help maintain the focus on the patient's desired goals while asking to share evidence-based interventions.

Treatment of Co-occurring Disorders

Patients with serious mental illness tend to have a higher prevalence of substance use, poorer treatment adherence, and worse health outcomes compared with the general population. Studies have suggested that pharmacotherapy for substance use disorders remains effective in this population (Roberts et al. 2015). Focusing on psychosocial interventions and treatment of co-occurring illness is important, especially when mental health care is being incorporated. As stated by the Substance Abuse and Mental Health Services Administration (Center for Substance Abuse Treatment 2005), the use of direct and transparent motivational interventions is one of the recommended approaches for treating patients with a co-occurring disorder.

EXAMPLE OF USE OF PHARMACOTHERAPY IN MOTIVATIONAL INTERVIEWING

> CLINICIAN: I understand that you would like to know more about medications to stop smoking cigarettes. Have you used anything to help you stop before? [*Elicit*]

TABLE 8–4. Medications for nicotine use disorder

Agent	FDA approval	Mechanism of action	Common side effects	Relative contraindications	Typical dosage and labs; comments
Nicotine replacement therapy: gum, patch, lozenge, oral inhaler, nasal spray	Beginning in 1984	Activates nicotinic receptors	Palpitations GI upset Insomnia (patch)	Severe cardiac disease Pregnancy Adolescence	2 mg/2 hours Combination is better than monotherapy; doses vary according to formulation used
Varenicline	2006	Nicotinic acetylcholine receptor partial agonist	Nausea Headache Insomnia	Severe neuropsychiatric symptoms	1 mg BID
Bupropion SR	1997	Norepinephrine and dopamine reuptake inhibitor Nicotinic acetylcholine receptor antagonist	Headache Dry mouth Insomnia	Epilepsy Eating disorder	150 mg BID

Note. This table is a summary only and is not meant to reflect a comprehensive review of the medications listed. GI=gastrointestinal.

PATIENT: I tried the patch, it didn't work. I just ended up smoking with it on, although less. I don't know that anything will work for me.

CLINICIAN: It's great that you tried to quit and are interested to try again. [*Affirmation*] Would it be okay if I shared some information that might be helpful? [*Ask permission*]

PATIENT: Yeah, sure.

CLINICIAN: The patch, which you know about, is part of a group of medications that replace nicotine. [*Building on patient knowledge*] In addition to the patch, there are shorter-acting medications, like the nicotine gum, lozenge, oral inhaler, and nasal spray. There are also two pills that are FDA-approved to help with quitting smoking, bupropion SR and varenicline. What do you know about these different options? [*Provide-elicit*]

PATIENT: I've tried the pills, but I was able to cut down more on the patch. Should I try it again?

CLINICIAN: Since nicotine replacement worked the best for you in the past but wasn't quite enough, I wonder if you would consider an increase the dose of nicotine you are getting? The different forms of nicotine replacement can be combined. [*Provide*]

PATIENT: Really? What do you mean?

CLINICIAN: You would keep the patch on all day, like last time. But when you're craving a cigarette, you could instead use the gum or any other of the short-acting nicotine medications. [*Provide*] What do you think about this combined approach? [*Elicit*]

PATIENT: Sure. I didn't realize I could use something else on top of the patch. I think having something I can take in the moment is going to make a huge difference.

KEY POINTS

- Motivational interviewing (MI) is a useful approach when incorporating pharmacotherapy into treatment.
    1. Engaging.
        a. Resist the assessment trap.
        b. Use open questions to discover what the patient understands to be the issue.
        c. Do not assume.
    2. Focusing.
        a. Identify the patient's goals and how medications align with achieving them.
        b. Build on information and experience from the past; collaborate on a plan for the future.

   c. Elicit what the patient knows about treatment. After asking permission, provide data about evidence-based treatment and medications in a transparent and factual manner. Elicit understanding and incorporation of newly provided information.

3. Evoking.

   a. Though medications are an important component of treatment and their utility is supported by evidence, there are many factors that limit their broad utilization.

   b. Appreciate that there are negatives to taking medications.

   c. Evoke change talk for taking medications.

   d. Support self-efficacy.

4. Planning.

   a. Offer a menu of options.

   b. Collaborate with the patient to formulate a plan of action for taking medication.

   c. Address barriers to treatment, help increase commitment to change, and continue to strengthen therapeutic alliance to increase adherence.

5. Support patient actions.

   a. Utilize evidence-based pharmacotherapies and provide information in a nonjudgmental, clear manner.

6. Ask about adherence.

   a. Use MI to foster an open discussion about potential issues of adherence, which are often complex and multifactorial.

   b. Acknowledge that adherence is difficult and periodically ask whether the patient is experiencing any problems taking his or her medication.

   c. Affirm any reduction of an undesired behavior and reflect upon it in the context of the patient's goals.

   d. If a patient experiences a return to use, use it as an opportunity to explore the patient's ambivalence rather than view it as a failure of treatment.

STUDY QUESTIONS

1. Why is motivational interviewing (MI) helpful in facilitating the use of medications?

    A. MI allows the patient to decide what they want to do, without the provider's input.
    B. It affords the opportunity to collaboratively build on information and experience from the past, leading to higher rates of success.
    C. It is not helpful in facilitating the use of medications in therapy.
    D. It allows the provider to list all of the reasons why the patient should take the medication, without interference with the patient's theoretical concerns.
    E. It allows the patient to be heard but ultimately relies on the provider's expertise to decide what is best.

2. After completing alcohol detoxification, a patient is interested in a medication to help him quit. He has never attempted to stop drinking before, but the need for hospitalization has really scared him. His laboratory results are significant for abnormally elevated liver function tests. Renal function is normal. What would you recommend?

    A. Disulfiram.
    B. Naltrexone.
    C. Acamprosate.
    D. Extended-release naltrexone.
    E. Alprazolam.

3. A patient says he wants to take medications to get better, but you call the pharmacy and discover he hasn't picked up his medications in months. What do you do?

    A. Nothing—see if he says anything at the next appointment.
    B. Discuss your discovery with the patient in a nonjudgmental and supportive way.
    C. Call the patient immediately and demand answers.
    D. Ask the patient to come in, ask open-ended questions, and, if he is amenable, restart medications with additional supports.
    E. Options B and D.

4. A patient has experienced a return to use of alcohol despite taking naltrexone and attending weekly therapy. What do you do?

A. Express your disappointment and ask the patient how she would like to proceed.

B. Call the patient's family.

C. Decide to no longer treat the patient, who probably wasn't really being compliant with the therapy, and refer her elsewhere.

D. Use the return as an opportunity to discuss triggers for relapse, and collaborate on next steps.

E. Tell the patient that this isn't working and that she has to go to a higher level of care.

5. A patient says that she has been using 120 mg of oxycodone daily for the past 2 years. She was initially prescribed oxycodone for a back injury but quickly began using more than prescribed. She says she would like to be detoxed. What is the next step?

A. Detox the patient.

B. Say you do not recommend detox and tell her you will only treat her with buprenorphine.

C. Refer the patient to a methadone clinic.

D. Ask, "What do you know about maintenance treatment for opioid addiction?"

E. Ask the patient how committed she is to treatment.

REFERENCES

Anderson R, Cissna KN: The Martin Buber–Carl Rogers Dialogue: A New Transcript With Commentary. Albany, State University of New York Press, 1997

Bandura A: Self-efficacy: toward a unifying theory of behavior change. Psychol Rev 84(2):191–215, 1977 847061

Center for Substance Abuse Treatment: Enhancing Motivation for Change in Substance Abuse Treatment (Treatment Improvement Protocol [TIP] Series No 35). Rockville, MD, Substance Abuse and Mental Health Services Administration, 1999

Center for Substance Abuse Treatment: Medication-Assisted Treatment for Opioid Addiction in Opioid Treatment Programs (Treatment Improvement Protocol [TIP] Series No 43). Rockville, MD, Substance Abuse and Mental Health Services Administration, 2005

Center for Substance Abuse Treatment: Incorporating Alcohol Pharmacotherapies Into Medical Practice (Treatment Improvement Protocol [TIP] Series No 49). Rockville, MD, Substance Abuse and Mental Health Services Administration, 2009

Centers for Disease Control and Prevention: Smoking and Tobacco Use, 2015. Available at: http://www.cdc.gov/tobacco/data_statistics/fact_sheets/fast_facts/index.htm. Accessed February 1, 2016.

Connery HS: Medication-assisted treatment of opioid use disorder: review of the evidence and future directions. Harv Rev Psychiatry 23(2):63–75, 2015 25747920

Dorr Goold S, Lipkin M Jr: The doctor-patient relationship: challenges, opportunities, and strategies. J Gen Intern Med 14(suppl 1):S26–S33, 1999 9933492

Jonas DE, Amick HR, Feltner C, et al: Pharmacotherapy for adults with alcohol use disorders in outpatient settings: a systematic review and meta-analysis. JAMA 311(18):1889–1900, 2014 24825644

Kranzler HR, Armeli S, Tennen H, et al: Targeted naltrexone for early problem drinkers. J Clin Psychopharmacol 23(3):294–304, 2003 12826991

Krueger KP, Berger BA, Felkey B: Medication adherence and persistence: a comprehensive review. Adv Ther 22(4):313–356, 2005 16418141

Magura S, Mateu PF, Rosenblum A, et al: Risk factors for medication non-adherence among psychiatric patients with substance misuse histories. Ment Health Subst Use 7(4):381–390, 2014 25309623

Mark TL, Kranzler HR, Poole VH, et al: Barriers to the use of medications to treat alcoholism. Am J Addict 12(4):281–294, 2003 14504021

Mark TL, Kassed CA, Vandivort-Warren R, et al: Alcohol and opioid dependence medications: prescription trends, overall and by physician specialty. Drug Alcohol Depend 99(1–3):345–349, 2009 18819759

Martin LR, Williams SL, Haskard KB, et al: The challenge of patient adherence. Ther Clin Risk Manag 1(3):189–199, 2005 18360559

Nieuwlaat R, Wilczynski N, Navarro T, et al: Interventions for enhancing medication adherence. Cochrane Database Syst Rev (11):CD000011, 2014 25412402

Roberts E, Evins AE, McNeill A, et al: Efficacy and acceptability of pharmacotherapy for smoking cessation in adults with serious mental illness: a systematic review and network meta-analysis. Addiction 111(4):599–612, 2015

Roman PM, Abraham AJ, Knudsen HK: Using medication-assisted treatment for substance use disorders: evidence of barriers and facilitators of implementation. Addict Behav 36(6):584–589, 2011 21377275

Stead LF, Perera R, Bullen C, et al: Nicotine replacement therapy for smoking cessation. Cochrane Database Syst Rev 11:CD000146, 2012 23152200

Substance Abuse and Mental Health Services Administration, Center for Behavioral Health Statistics and Quality: Treatment Episode Data Set (TEDS): 2000–2010. National Admissions to Substance Abuse Treatment Services. DASIS Series S-61, HHS Publication No (SMA) 12-4701. Rockville, MD, Substance Abuse and Mental Health Services Administration, 2012

Talwar A, Jain M, Vijayan VK: Pharmacotherapy of tobacco dependence. Med Clin North Am 88(6):1517–1534, 2004 15464111

Willey C: Behavior-changing methods for improving adherence to medication. Curr Hypertens Rep 1(6):477–481, 1999 10981109

STUDENT REFLECTIONS

Emmanuel Ohuabunwa, M.D., M.B.A. candidate
Yale School of Medicine, MS4

As a future emergency medicine practitioner, and having seen the sheer numbers of patients presenting each day with acute exacerbations of substance use disorders, I read this chapter with excitement at its relevance to my future practice. The most important broken myth was the idea that using motivational interviewing (MI) takes too much time and is therefore not relevant in the emergency room (ER). With the techniques suggested, I learned that the ER physician pressed for time could at least broach the subject to his or her patients, ascertain their willingness to change, and bring in appropriate providers to the ER depending on the patients' preference. The presentation of a structured approach to these conversations in time-constrained settings, such as the "elicit-provide-elicit" framework, with specific examples, really reinforces its utility. The authors also warned of potential pitfalls providers are prone to, including assessment and expert traps and ways to deal with them, the most important of which are ensuring shared decision making and approaching patients in a nonjudgmental manner. Another important topic that was explored concerns the potential for pharmacotherapy to replace the intrinsic motivations of an addicted patient, leading to less than optimal results. The chapter suggests that providers can avoid this by constantly probing the patient's motivations and maintaining an open, nonjudgmental line of communication. I especially liked the charts outlining the most common medications used, their mechanisms of action, and the types of patients for which each medication is recommended. If such charts are not already available in a readily accessible format, I would love for these to be placed on laminated cards that physicians can carry in their lab coats. Overall, I've learned a lot about the ways to approach pharmacotherapy for patients with addiction, potential pitfalls to avoid, and techniques to increase the likelihood of success.

Motivational Interviewing in a Diverse Society

Brian Hurley, M.D., M.B.A., DFASAM
Jeffrey DeVido, M.D., M.T.S.

> Differences simply act as a yarn of curiosity unraveling until we get to
> the other side.
>
> —*Ciore Taylor*

Researchers have studied the use of motivational interviewing (MI) in numerous clinical settings, from emergency departments, outpatient medical settings, and substance use treatment programs to inpatient medical and surgical units, dental offices, and even classrooms. Much of the research has been organized around either specific diagnostic entities, such as alcohol and opioid use disorders, or specific target behaviors, such as diet modification in individuals with diabetes or medication adherence. Comparatively little research on the effectiveness and application of MI has been organized around patient- or clientspecific factors such as nationality, culture, age, race and ethnicity, sexual orientation, gender, or religious or spiritual preference or affiliation. The question remains, therefore, whether there are particular patient- or client-specific factors worth considering in the decision to employ MI, or how one might tailor an intervention based on these factors. In this chapter, we review the available literature on MI in relation to these diverse patient- or client-specific factors. On the basis of these data, we provide examples of implementation of MI in a patient- or client-specific manner, along with some additional tips for consideration with these patient or client specific-factors in mind.

COUNTRIES AND LANGUAGES

While certainly not synonymous with the entire diversity of patient- or client-specific factors one may encounter (such as culture, race, or ethnicity), the array of different nations and languages in which MI has been or is being implemented may at least provide a sense of the geographic range of MI's reach. The Motivational Interviewing Network of Trainers (MINT), for example, is a global organization aimed at connecting clinicians who are actively engaged in training others in the skills of MI, and their website (www.motivationalinterviewing.org/trainer-listing) currently lists trainers in at least 30 different countries. The foundational MI book authored by William Miller and Stephen Rollnick, *Motivational Interviewing: Helping People Change*, now in its third edition (Miller and Rollnick 2013), is available in 9 different languages, and overall books relating to MI can be found in at least 19 different languages. While the majority of the literature has been published from English-speaking countries, studies on MI have been undertaken throughout the world in multiple languages. To date, there is little to suggest that MI would not be applicable in any particular region or in any particular language. However, the global expansion of access to MI educational materials, mentoring, and research base will undoubtedly help increase our understanding of 1) how applicable this engagement technique is across different nations and languages, and 2) whether specific skills or approaches may be worth considering when employing MI in different languages and/or countries/regions.

AGE

Studies of MI have demonstrated its utility not only in adult populations but also on the opposite ends of the age spectrum: pediatric/adolescent and geriatric populations.

Researchers have published several hundred studies on MI in pediatric/adolescent populations for a range of disorders and behavioral targets, including substance use disorders, obesity prevention and management, and medication adherence (especially in type 1 diabetes). Data have generally supported the notion that MI can be effective in positively altering adolescent behavior. A 2014 meta-analysis of the literature, for example, looking specifically at MI efficacy in modulating adolescent non-substance-using behavior, demonstrated a small, but significant, post-intervention effect compared with control subjects (Cushing et al. 2014). Data pertaining to the efficacy of MI for substance use disorders in pediatric/adolescent populations have been mixed. On the one hand, a 2014 Cochrane systematic review included 66 randomized control trials of MI for alcohol misuse disorders and concluded that "there are no substantive, meaningful benefits of MI interventions for the prevention of alcohol misuse" (Foxcroft et al. 2014). However, the authors acknowledged heterogeneity and potential biases in the dataset or analysis, respectively, that could account for those findings. Moreover, this review was withdrawn from the databank in 2015, citing errors in the review. Other studies, however, have demonstrated significant effects on substance use behaviors in pediatric/adolescent populations in various venues: psychiatric emergency (Bagoien et al. 2013) and medical emergency settings (Cunningham et al. 2015), substance-specific treatment groups (marijuana) (D'Amico et al. 2015), and first-time legal offender programs (D'Amico et al. 2013). It stands to reason, on the one hand, that the pediatric/adolescent population, ripe with developmentally appropriate ambivalence and frustration, may benefit from an MI approach, given that such an approach aims to normalize both ambivalence and resistance. On the other hand, one could reason that adolescents do not have stable identity or behavioral patterns, and may have more difficulty sustaining healthful behavioral changes. Further data will undoubtedly clarify this conundrum.

Comparatively fewer studies have looked specifically at geriatric populations. A 2009 literature review by Cummings and colleagues (2009) summarized 15 studies demonstrating the effectiveness of MI in elderly patients for a range of target behaviors, including improved physical activity, diet, cholesterol, blood pressure, and glycemic control, and increased rate of smoking cessation. One included study even demonstrated the effectiveness of MI applied to work with geriatric clients over the telephone (Kolt et al. 2007). However, in their 2009 review, Cummings and colleagues remarked that the effects of MI interventions appear to be short-lived and the included studies tended to be small, with little demographic diversity (predominantly Caucasian), and relied on self-reported outcomes, which may limit the generalizability of these findings. In a separate publication, researchers highlighted a strategy they employed for combining cognitive-behavioral therapy (CBT) and MI to address alcohol and other substance use behaviors in elderly men and women (Cooper 2012). The authors indicated that they consciously incorporated "aging specific consequences of using alcohol or other substances [such as educational information about the unique health risks posed by substance use to the geriatric population]" into their use of MI in this population, with good effect. This finding may hint at broader mechanisms for both acknowledging and operationalizing patient- or client-specific factors in MI.

These data reflect the data on MI as a whole; namely, there is a wide degree of variability in MI outcomes in both the pediatric/adolescent and geriatric populations, and further studies are necessary to determine the full effect of MI in these populations. However, in both populations a key point is highlighted: acknowledging the broader social and developmental background in which a patient or client sits can be an important tool for most effectively engaging in MI.

RACE AND ETHNICITY

For the purposes of this book, *race* refers to a person's physical characteristics (such as skin color), while *ethnicity* refers to cultural factors (such as language, nationality, regional cultural practices). A person's race and ethnicity can both be significantly important to how a person self-identifies and may therefore contribute to core values that the person may hold. Behavioral interventions, in general, may need to be adapted to account for cultural differences, especially when evidence-based treatments are not working for a particular group (Lakes et al. 2006; López and Guarnaccia 2000). It stands to reason, therefore, that appreciation, identification, and incorporation of aspects of a person's race and ethnicity into an MI encounter may help facilitate engagement and foster a deeper conversation regarding values that could lead to greater change talk and consequent better behavioral outcomes. Although there is an emerging literature in this area, further research is needed to validate or refute this notion.

There is some evidence to suggest that better attention to ethnic matching of provider and patient/client can yield better clinical outcomes. A 2005 U.S.-based meta-analysis found that MI effects were larger for ethnic minority populations, especially Native American groups, which the authors suggested may be because "the client-centered, supportive, and non-confrontational style of MI may resemble the normative communication style of Indian populations, at least in the American Southwest, thereby representing a culturally congruent intervention" (Hettema et al. 2005). Additionally, Field and Caetano (2010) provided a brief MI intervention for Hispanic patients or clients ($N=537$) who presented to a trauma center with injuries related to alcohol use disorder. The brief interventions were conducted by either Hispanic providers or non-Hispanic providers. The authors determined that Hispanic patients or clients matched ethnically with Hispanic providers did better at 12-month follow-up relative to their unmatched cohorts. Field et al. (2015) are now examining this phenomenon in a larger, more specific study. One theory they have proposed in order to explain their findings is that certain shared cultural experiences shared by members of the same community (such as familyism and acculturation challenges in the Hispanic community) are conveyed implicitly through "culturally appropriate modes of communication" (Field et al. 2015, p. 2).

Researchers have examined the efficacy of MI for a number of behavioral targets in the African American community, with mixed results. MI, for example, failed to show benefit in a weight loss program for obese African American women (Befort et al. 2008), but it has shown significant benefits in other studies. For example, in one study, African American individuals with type 2 diabetes who were exposed to MI had significantly lower glucose levels and body mass index and better exercise adherence (race or ethnicity of provider of study intervention was not specified) (Chlebowy et al. 2015). Other studies have similarly demonstrated the efficacy of MI in African American populations for antihypertensive medication adherence (Ogedegbe et al. 2008) and in African American adolescents for asthma medication adherence (Riekert et al. 2011).

Native Americans are known to be disproportionately affected by substance use disorders, and providing culturally appropriate prevention and intervention or treatment programs is challenging but necessary. As previously alluded to, there are emerging data looking at the incorporation of MI in Native American populations. A secondary analysis of a large study of psychotherapies for alcohol use disorder found that Native American participants responded better to motivational enhancement therapy than to CBT or 12-step facilitation therapy. Additionally, Venner et al. (2008) developed a culturally adapted MI manual specific to Native American groups that grew out of focus groups that explored unique communication patterns for negotiating change in these communities. The authors made several culture-specific recommendations for using MI with Native American clients. Among these recommendations were that providers 1) be careful not to stereotype; 2) introduce themselves fully, including specifying what languages they speak, and tell a bit about their parents and family; 3) don't ask specifics about spiritual practices, because many of these are private and sacred; 4) be aware of historical traumas; and 5) learn about specific cultures and cultural practices of the group with whom they are interfacing. In a similarly focused effort, Dickerson et al. (2016) developed a strategy for incorporating appreciation of traditional Native American cultural practices and beliefs with Native American youths in urban settings. The authors specifically highlighted that many Native American youths, through historical trauma related to relocation or forced relocation, feel disconnected with their cultural heritage. Through incorporation of beading, prayer or sage ceremony, and cooking into the traditional MI format for substance use disorders, the authors reported being able to better engage these youths.

Overall, the role played by race and ethnicity in the efficacy of MI is understudied. However, an emerging literature across several different ethnic and racial groups suggests that ethnic and racial factors can play a significant role in the efficacy of MI. Specifically, in Hispanic populations, researchers have shown better efficacy when MI is delivered by a provider of similar Hispanic background. Specific similar effects have not been documented in other racial and ethnic populations, although there also are no documented trials of such. In Native American populations, researchers have demonstrated increased efficacy when traditional practices are incorporated with conventional MI conversations. These data reaffirm 1) the importance of the provider-patient relationship and the finding that even subtle cultural familiarities and nonverbal cues can be powerfully beneficial in eliciting change, and 2) the versatility of MI as a flexible medium that can be stretched and molded creatively to take into account a range of patient- or client-specific factors, such as ethnicity and race.

LESBIAN, GAY, BISEXUAL, AND TRANSGENDER

The diversity of sexual orientations, gender identities, gender expressions, and sex development along the spectrum of human experiences are as vast as the number of people in the world. In general, *sexual orientation* typically refers to erotic arousal and attraction and itself has behavioral, expressed identity, and internal feeling components. *Gender identity* refers to one's internal identification with a gender, and the term *transgender* generally refers to the adoption of a gender identity different from the gender assigned at birth. *Gender expression* comprises the behavioral traits, clothing choices, and other markers that communicate a person's gender, which may or may not confirm to societal norms. *Sex development* is the aggregate of biological traits that create differences along the male-female anatomical and physiological spectrum. These domains each function independently of one another, apply to every human being, and provide a foundation for understanding that not all people share the same sexual orientations, gender identities, gender expressions, and sex development (Shively and De Cecco 1977).

Heterosexism, homophobia, and transphobia serve to stigmatize the experience of people who identify as lesbian, gay, bisexual (DiPlacido 1998), and transgender (Hendricks and Testa 2012). As such, lesbian, gay, bisexual, transgender (LGBT) populations experience distinct health disparities, and optimal care therefore requires clinicians to be aware of and sensitive to "historical stigmatization, to be informed about continued barriers to care and the differential prevalence of specific risk factors and health conditions in these populations, and to become aware of the cultural aspects of their interactions with LGBT patients" (Mayer et al. 2008, p. 990).

Within this context, MI can be considered an ideal method to engage people who may identify as LGBT, given the technique's emphasis on partnership, acceptance (including autonomy), compassion, and evocation. In an MI encounter, the clinician accepts a stance of curiosity, which can help avoid making misplaced assumptions about the sexual orientation or gender identity of the patient/client with whom he or she may be working. All clinicians work with people who identify as LGBT, so maintaining openness optimizes care for people of all sexual orientations, gender identities, gender expressions, and sex development. Notably, there is nothing in the literature to suggest that men, women, or people with any other gender respond differentially to MI.

Research on MI in LGBT populations has had a dominant focus on gay and bisexual men. There are multiple studies showing that MI has some effectiveness in reducing HIV risk behaviors in men who have sex with men (Chariyeva et al. 2012; Harding et al. 2001; Naar-King et al. 2006; Parsons et al. 2014; Rutledge et al. 2001). There is additional research that MI can be effective at reducing alcohol use among men who have sex with men who have alcohol use disorders (Morgenstern et al. 2007). Studies are not uniformly positive for all outcomes studied, and a meta-analysis suggested that MI's effect on HIV risk behaviors among men who have sex with men may be modest at best (Berg et al. 2011). One critique of this meta-analysis and the many negative studies is that the fidelity to the MI technique was not factored into the study analysis. A more recent review of four meta-analyses has found MI to be a generally effective treatment to reduce risky behaviors and increase patient or client engagement (Lundahl and Burke 2009).

There is little research looking specifically at the effect of MI when working with lesbian or bisexual women, but there is nothing to suggest that lesbian or bisexual women would benefit differentially from MI techniques. A study of homeless youths that included lesbian and bisexual adolescents found that youths who received MI had reduced illicit drug use (other than marijuana) compared with a control group, but this study was not powered to study MI's effect on the subsample of lesbian and bisexual adolescents (Peterson et al. 2006). Given that there is evidence that lesbian and bisexual women are at risk for hazardous alcohol use and alcohol-related problems (Green and Feinstein 2012), there are opportunities to apply MI to address alcohol-related behaviors in lesbian and bisexual women. Overall, MI is a standard evidence-based practice described when authors discuss the clinical approach to LGBT populations that include both lesbian and bisexual women (Anderson 2009).

Research on health practices improving the health of transgender and gender-nonconforming populations is sparse. There is a conceptual model supporting clinical work with patients who are transgender or gender nonconforming that relies heavily on MI, and this supports that MI may be as useful when working with transgender people as it is with cisgender populations (Hendricks and Testa 2012). MI's spirit is based on the principles of partnership, acceptance (including autonomy), compassion, and evocation—all of which will serve clinicians well in working with transgender and gender-nonconforming patients/clients.

MI is congruent with the fundamentals of working with LGBT populations. Good clinicians should be reasonably free of homophobia, transphobia, and heterosexism; have positive regard for the patient; welcome and promote openness about sexual orientation and gender identity in the therapeutic setting; and be familiar with many of the issues commonly faced by LGBT people (Lee 2015).

EXAMPLES OF USE OF MOTIVATIONAL INTERVIEWING IN A DIVERSE SOCIETY

MI occurs in four phases—engaging, focusing, evoking, and planning—which can be used in the following ways to address diverse populations.

Engaging

- Determining which gender pronouns a patient/client wants to use.
- Learning a patient's or client's age, religion, gender, and national origin.
- Discussing patient/client understandings of health and risk behaviors (which are culturally informed).
- Exploring the extent of clinician–patient or –client alliance and/or discord, which may be driven by cultural differences.
- Remaining open to learning a patient's/client's cultural background, sexual orientation, and/or gender identity, if the patient/client chooses to discuss it.

Focusing

- Partnering with patients on mutually agreeable behaviors to address, in light of culturally informed patient- or client-defined understandings of health and risk behaviors.

Evoking

- Understanding the extent to which one's experience with age-specific or developmental stage differences, racism, sexism, trauma, homophobia, inner or externalized conflicts, or internal comfort with identity shapes decision making about health behaviors.

Planning

- Planning in a culturally responsive approach where decision making is shared with and defined by the patient/client. This approach inherently incorporates the intersectionality of the patient's/client's identities, understandings, and beliefs.

USE OF MOTIVATIONAL INTERVIEWING IN STRUCTURALLY COMPETENT CARE

There are structural-level determinants of health that generate health disparities based on race, culture, ethnicity, sexual orientation, gender, and gender identity. Addressing these structural-level determinants is referred to as *structural competency* (Hansen and Metzl 2016). Cross et al. (1989) identified five core concepts of cultural (and structural) competence in a system: value of diversity, cultural self-assessment, consciousness of the dynamics of cultural interaction, institutionalization of cultural knowledge, and adaptations to diversity. These core elements are resonant with the appropriate application of MI. Table 9–1 delineates the application of MI principles along the five concepts of structural competence.

TABLE 9–1. Use of motivational interviewing (MI) in structurally competent care

Structurally competent concept	MI application
Value diversity	Valuing diversity is supported by MI's spirit of autonomy and patient- or client-centered style.
Conduct self-assessment	Reflections used during the course of MI serve as a check on the clinician's assumptions and require mindfulness in the clinician. Discord in the relationship requires that clinicians change behavior.
Manage the dynamics of difference	Dynamics of difference can be managed by MI's spirit of acceptance, including autonomy, and partnership despite differences.
Acquire and incorporate cultural knowledge	MI evokes patient- or client-based goals, values, and understandings.
Adapt to the diversity and cultural context of the individuals whom clinicians serve	The focusing and planning phases require shared decision making and benefit from a shared understanding of cultural context. The use of reflections requires adaptations to patient/client input informed by cultural context.

KEY POINTS

- Motivational interviewing (MI) is used throughout the world in numerous languages.

- There is robust evidence to support the effectiveness of MI in adolescents, and some evidence to suggest that MI has some positive effect in geriatric populations.

- There is some evidence to suggest that racial/ethnic concordance of the MI clinician and patient/client enhances the efficacy of MI.

- MI that judiciously incorporates cultural norms can improve the engagement phase of the interview.

- There is no evidence that MI has more or less effect in lesbian, gay, bisexual, and transgender (LGBT) patients than in the general population.

- MI's emphasis on partnership, acceptance (including autonomy), compassion, and evocation supports clinicians working with LGBT patients, where openness can help avoid misplaced assumptions.

- Good clinicians should be reasonably free of homophobia, transphobia, and heterosexism; have positive regard for the patient; welcome and promote openness about sexual orientation and gender identity in the therapeutic setting; and be familiar with many of the issues commonly faced by LGBT persons.

- MI is congruent with structurally competent care.

STUDY QUESTIONS

1. How would you best describe the evidence that motivational interviewing (MI) supports adolescents changing their drug- or alcohol-related behaviors?

    A. The evidence is mixed (some studies show an effect, and other studies show no effect.

    B. The evidence is consistently positive (a strong positive effect).

    C. The evidence shows overwhelming harm (a strong detrimental effect).

    D. The evidence consistently shows no effect on drug or alcohol use in adolescents.

2. How does the effect of MI with racial and ethnic minorities in the United States compare with the effect shown in the general population?

    A. MI has been shown to be more harmful to racial and ethnic minorities.

    B. MI has been shown to have a stronger positive effect with racial and ethnic minorities.

C. MI consistently works no better or worse.

D. MI always requires the patient/client and clinician to be of the same race/ethnicity to show any benefit.

3. In which of the following situations was MI shown to have the strongest effect?

A. When Native Americans are asked directly about their spiritual practices.

B. When African American patients/clients are working with African American clinicians.

C. When the clinician and patient/client share subtle cultural familiarities and nonverbal cues.

D. When MI is provided in strict accordance with a manual.

4. What has the majority of MI research involving gay and bisexual men focused on?

A. Cigarette smoking.

B. Eating behaviors.

C. Alcohol use.

D. HIV risk behaviors.

5. Determining which gender pronouns a patient/client identifies with is part of which phase of MI?

A. Engaging.

B. Focusing.

C. Evoking.

D. Planning.

REFERENCES

Anderson SC: Substance Use Disorders in Lesbian, Gay, Bisexual, and Transgender Clients: Assessment and Treatment. New York, Columbia University Press, 2009

Bagoien G, Bjorngaard JH, Ostensen C, et al: The effects of motivational interviewing on patients with comorbid substance use admitted to a psychiatric emergency unit—a randomised controlled trial with two year follow-up. BMC Psychiatry 13:93, 2013

Befort CA, Nollen N, Ellerbeck EF, et al: Motivational interviewing fails to improve outcomes of a behavioral weight loss program for obese African American women: a pilot randomized trial. J Behav Med 31(5):367–377, 2008 18587639

Berg RC, Ross MW, Tikkanen R: The effectiveness of MI4MSM: how useful is motivational interviewing as an HIV risk prevention program for men who have sex with men? A systematic review. AIDS Educ Prev 23(6):533–549, 2011 22201237

Chariyeva Z, Golin CE, Earp JA, et al: Does motivational interviewing counseling time influence HIV-positive persons' self-efficacy to practice safer sex? Patient Educ Couns 87(1):101–107, 2012 21890300

Chlebowy DO, El-Mallakh P, Myers J, et al: Motivational interviewing to improve diabetes outcomes in African Americans adults with diabetes. West J Nurs Res 37(5):566–580, 2015 24733233

Cooper L: Combined motivational interviewing and cognitive–behavioral therapy with older adult drug and alcohol abusers. Health Soc Work 37(3):173–179, 2012

Cross T, Bazron B, Dennis K, Isaacs M: Towards a Culturally Competent System of Care, Vol I. Washington, DC, Georgetown University Child Development Center, CASSP Technical Assistance Center, 1989

Cummings SM, Cooper RL, Cassie KM: Motivational interviewing to affect behavioral change in older adults. Res Soc Work Pract 19(2):195–204, 2009

Cunningham RM, Chermack ST, Ehrlich PF, et al: Alcohol interventions among underage drinkers in the ED: a randomized controlled trial. Pediatrics 136(4):e783–e793, 2015 26347440

Cushing CC, Jensen CD, Miller MB, et al: Meta-analysis of motivational interviewing for adolescent health behavior: efficacy beyond substance use. J Consult Clin Psychol 82(6):1212–1218, 2014 24841861

D'Amico EJ, Hunter SB, Miles JN, et al: A randomized controlled trial of a group motivational interviewing intervention for adolescents with a first time alcohol or drug offense. J Subst Abuse Treat 45(5):400–408, 2013 23891459

D'Amico EJ, Houck JM, Hunter SB, et al: Group motivational interviewing for adolescents: change talk and alcohol and marijuana outcomes. J Consult Clin Psychol 83(1):68–80, 2015 25365779

Dickerson DL, Brown RA, Johnson CL, et al: Integrating motivational interviewing and traditional practices to address alcohol and drug use among urban American Indian/Alaska Native youth. J Subst Abuse Treat 65:26–35, 2016 26306776

DiPlacido J: Minority Stress Among Lesbians, Gay Men, and Bisexuals: A Consequence of Heterosexism, Homophobia, and Stigmatization. Thousand Oaks, CA, Sage, 1998

Field C, Caetano R: The role of ethnic matching between patient and provider on the effectiveness of brief alcohol interventions with Hispanics. Alcohol Clin Exp Res 34(2):262–271, 2010 19951297

Field CA, Cabriales JA, Woolard RH, et al: Cultural adaptation of a brief motivational intervention for heavy drinking among Hispanics in a medical setting. BMC Public Health 15:724, 2015 26223781

Foxcroft DR, Coombes L, Wood S, et al: Motivational interviewing for alcohol misuse in young adults. Cochrane Database Syst Rev 8(8):CD007025, 2014 25140980

Green KE, Feinstein BA: Substance use in lesbian, gay, and bisexual populations: an update on empirical research and implications for treatment. Psychol Addict Behav 26(2):265–278, 2012 22061339

Hansen H, Metzl J: Structural competency in the US healthcare crisis: putting social and policy interventions into clinical practice. Journal of Bioethical Inquiry 13:1–5, 2016

Harding R, Dockrell MJ, Dockrell J, et al: Motivational interviewing for HIV risk reduction among gay men in commercial and public sex settings. AIDS Care 13(4):493–501, 2001 11454270

Hendricks ML, Testa RJ: A conceptual framework for clinical work with transgender and gender nonconforming clients: An adaptation of the Minority Stress Model. Prof Psychol Res Pr 43(5):460–467, 2012

Hettema J, Steele J, Miller WR: Motivational interviewing. Annu Rev Clin Psychol 1:91–111, 2005

Kolt GS, Schofield GM, Kerse N, et al: Effect of telephone counseling on physical activity for low-active older people in primary care: a randomized, controlled trial. J Am Geriatr Soc 55(7):986–992, 2007 17608869

Lakes K, López SR, Garro LC: Cultural competence and psychotherapy: applying anthropologically informed conceptions of culture. Psychotherapy (Chic) 43(4):380–396, 2006 22122131

Lee SJ: Addiction and lesbian, gay, bisexual and transgender (LGBT) issues, in Textbook of Addiction Treatment: International Perspectives. Edited by el-Guebaly N, Carrà G, Galanter M. New York, Springer, 2015, pp 2139–2164

López SR, Guarnaccia PJ: Cultural psychopathology: uncovering the social world of mental illness. Annu Rev Psychol 51(1):571–598, 2000 10751981

Lundahl B, Burke BL: The effectiveness and applicability of motivational interviewing: a practice-friendly review of four meta-analyses. J Clin Psychol 65(11):1232–1245, 2009 19739205

Mayer KH, Bradford JB, Makadon HJ, et al: Sexual and gender minority health: what we know and what needs to be done. Am J Public Health 98(6):989–995, 2008 18445789

Miller WR, Rollnick S: Motivational Interviewing: Helping People Change, 3rd Edition. New York, Guilford, 2013

Morgenstern J, Irwin TW, Wainberg ML, et al: A randomized controlled trial of goal choice interventions for alcohol use disorders among men who have sex with men. J Consult Clin Psychol 75(1):72–84, 2007 17295566

Naar-King S, Wright K, Parsons JT, et al: Healthy choices: motivational enhancement therapy for health risk behaviors in HIV-positive youth. AIDS Educ Prev 18(1):1–11, 2006 16539572

Ogedegbe G, Chaplin W, Schoenthaler A, et al: A practice-based trial of motivational interviewing and adherence in hypertensive African Americans. Am J Hypertens 21(10):1137–1143, 2008 18654123

Parsons JT, Lelutiu-Weinberger C, Botsko M, et al: A randomized controlled trial utilizing motivational interviewing to reduce HIV risk and drug use in young gay and bisexual men. J Consult Clin Psychol 82(1):9–18, 2014 24364800

Peterson PL, Baer JS, Wells EA, et al: Short-term effects of a brief motivational intervention to reduce alcohol and drug risk among homeless adolescents. Psychol Addict Behav 20(3):254–264, 2006 16938063

Riekert KA, Borrelli B, Bilderback A, et al: The development of a motivational interviewing intervention to promote medication adherence among inner-city, African-American adolescents with asthma. Patient Educ Couns 82(1):117–122, 2011 20371158

Rutledge SE, Roffman RA, Mahoney C, et al: Motivational enhancement counseling strategies in delivering a telephone-based brief HIV prevention intervention. Clin Soc Work J 29(3):291–306, 2001

Shively MG, De Cecco JP: Components of sexual identity. J Homosex 3(1):41–48, 1977 591712

Venner KL, Feldstein SW, Tafoya N: Helping clients feel welcome: principles of adapting treatment cross-culturally. Alcohol Treat Q 25(4):11–30, 2008 20671813

STUDENT REFLECTIONS

David Kopel
Rutgers New Jersey Medical School, MS-IV

Patient diversity colors every physician's clinical interactions but is often over-looked by even the most conscientious providers. Acknowledgment and response to diversity take active effort on the part of the provider; that is, it is insufficient to merely reject malignant biases like racism and transphobia. Rather, inclusive health care requires the physician to recognize the relevance of diversity to individual clinical scenarios and respond appropriately. Particularly in the context of motivational interviewing (MI), trust is paramount. The findings in this chapter provide both reassurance and a challenge to practitioners.

The tactics and values inherent in effective MI can be applied to a wide variety of ages and backgrounds. One need not fear that an elderly or homosexual patient, for instance, will not benefit from effective MI. On the other hand, the finding that familiarity with LGBTQ issues creates an atmosphere of trust puts the burden on doctors to learn about these issues, whether they be the preferred pronouns of their patients, the specific kinds of violence faced by the trans community or the indications for the use of pre-exposure HIV prophylaxis. Of particular interest is the existence of evidence to substantiate the idea that racial/ethnic concordance between provider and patient increases the efficacy of MI. This issue deserves further investigation before its implications are fully clear, but preliminarily it may provide some support to doctors who make a conscious effort to hire a diverse staff or at the very least to educate themselves about a wide variety of cultural practices and norms. Ultimately, compassion and respect remain the cornerstones of effective therapeutic relationships, but this chapter highlights the need to translate those values into active efforts to learn about culture.

Getting Advanced Knowledge in Motivational Interviewing

Teaching Motivational Interviewing

Carla Marienfeld, M.D.
Caridad C. Ponce Martinez, M.D.
Curtis Bone, M.D., M.H.S.

> Tell me and I forget. Teach me and I remember. Involve me and I learn.
>
> —*Benjamin Franklin*

> Teaching is more than imparting knowledge, it is inspiring change. Learning is more than absorbing facts, it is acquiring skills.
>
> —*William Arthur Ward*

In this chapter we provide practical teaching strategies using the frame of the four motivational interviewing (MI) processes (engaging, focusing, evoking, and planning) and example content to use. Teaching strategies include didactic and experiential learning followed by supervision, monitoring, and feedback. The goal is for these strategies to recapitulate the spirit of MI.

To begin, let's consider our thoughts and approaches to teaching psychotherapy. What are the qualities of an ineffective teacher? What are the qualities of an effective teacher? These are not rhetorical questions; rather, they are MI-inspired open questions intended to engage you in thinking about teaching MI. Allow us to share some thoughts about ineffective and effective teachers that may augment your own thoughts (in the absence of an ability to solicit responses from you, the readers, we'll substitute the paraphrased results from a quick Internet search). Ineffective teachers do not allow for growth and change (critical to MI!) or allow education from the student; they prevent or dismiss individual problem solving and innovative ideas, have a limited view of the student or topic, use methods that suit the teacher rather than the student, lack initiative or motivation to change and adapt teaching, and lack insight about their limited effectiveness. Effective teachers, on the other hand, engage students, possess the capacity for adaptation, present clear learning objectives, clearly communicate ideas and knowledge, commit to the student, expect the best from students, work collaboratively, possess a good balance between confidence and humility, and convey passion, knowledge, and rapport.

Goals in teaching MI include effectively conveying the spirit, processes, and skills of MI and helping learners to be competent practitioners of MI. How do you plan to be an effective teacher? How will you know if you have taught MI well?

In this chapter, MI teaching strategies are presented through the four processes. Examples are offered of concrete teaching strategies that may enhance student participation and motivation throughout training sessions. In addition, a frame informed by the Gradual Release of Responsibility Model—commonly understood as the "I do it, we do it, you do it" model (Frey et al. 2009)—is also a way of approaching the instruction of MI that can be consistent with the MI style.

- "I do it." MODELING. The teacher introduces the skill, role-models the skill, provides examples, and demonstrates use.
- "We do it." COLLABORATION/MONITORING. The teacher participates with trainees in practicing skills; trainees practice the skill in a small group, with the trainer leading the exercise; and trainees role-play among themselves, with the trainer listening and offering information and advice as appropriate.
- "You do it." SUPERVISION/FEEDBACK. Trainees are allowed time for independent practice and making mistakes. The trainer observes (in real time or after) use of the skills, solicits trainee input about the experience, reflects trainee feedback to the trainee, affirms skills well executed, and offers summaries. The trainer can also offer observations and opportunities for improvement as appropriate.

Examples: Open Questions

"I do it." The teacher can start with a definition and examples of open questions. He or she is thus modeling how to differentiate open questions from closed questions.

"We do." The teacher then allows trainees to participate in the differentiation of open questions from closed questions. Offer information and assistance is provided as needed.

"I do it." The teacher can model how to transform closed questions into open questions.

"You do it." The teacher can ask the trainees to provide examples of closed questions and can allow the group to transform them into open questions. The class can split into pairs and practice turning each other's closed questions into open questions while the teacher listens and provides feedback. The same process can be applied to affirming, reflecting, and summarizing.

Let's take a moment to more fully explore the "we do" component of this skills training model and to introduce a few concrete teaching strategies. Most facilitators are comfortable with offering instruction or modeling a skill (the "I do" component) and requesting independent practice (the "you do" component); however, many struggle with soliciting participation in the group setting (the "we do" component). It can be difficult to comfortably enlist participation in a group setting, even when teaching motivated adult learners. Nevertheless, this piece of skills training remains essential, because it is an opportunity for everyone to learn from mistakes and establish comfort before working independently. It also allows for more independent role-play. Varying the method of interaction can enrich comfort and enjoyment with group practice. A few examples of strategies include "round-robin," "popcorn style," "fishbowl technique," and "tag team." By varying the style of interaction during group practice, the learners are more likely to remain attentive and involved. The more learners are involved, the higher likelihood they will acquire the desired skills during group practice. This will further enhance the utility of independent practice during which learners reinforce and refine their understanding of each technique.

Example: OARS

When teaching OARS (**o**pen questions, **a**ffirmations, **r**eflections, **s**ummaries), after students independently practice asking open questions, the facilitator might move on to discussing affirmations. The facilitator might begin with a statement, "I just can't quit smoking. I keep trying, but I can't beat it." In the "I do" component of teaching, the facilitator will model how one might affirm this statement, saying "You keep trying. You haven't given up. That shows a lot of strength and fortitude." For group practice of "we do," an option would be to request individuals from the class to also complete this task.

Soliciting a volunteer to participate can lead to an awkward silence and discomfort. Another option would be to inform the class that everyone will be asked to take a turn (if it is a relatively small class) and do a round-robin. Everyone in the room practices an affirmation to a statement; though if the group is large, the facilitator might select a smaller defined subset of the group. When teaching another skill, during the "we do" phase of skill training, the facilitator could opt for popcorn questions. The facilitator bounces from person to person at random, eliciting participation. This can be done simply by calling names, pointing, or drawing names from a cup. A different popcorn style technique involves the use of a ball. The moderator can throw the ball to the first student volunteer. The student then throws the ball to a fellow student who becomes the next volunteer. This can continue on until the facilitator requests the ball back and concludes the exercise. Fishbowl practice is ideal for longer role-plays and is commonly used when teaching reflections and summaries. The entire class watches two individuals participate in a role-play. The facilitator then times out the role-play intermittently and solicits input from the class to coach the physician and/or the patient in the case. Using the tag-team technique, the class instructor acts as the patient and four students function as a tag team during the encounter. It begins with the first student, who offers an open question followed by an instructor response. The second student offers an affirmation followed by an instructor response. The third student offers a reflection followed by an instructor response, and then the fourth student offers a summary.

TEACHING THE SPIRIT OF MOTIVATIONAL INTERVIEWING

During MI training, we are asking participants to change a behavior (the way they interact with patients), to not be locked into the expert role, and to learn a different way of being with and talking to patients. Therefore, adoption of the MI spirit on the part of the trainer is desirable for change to occur.

Let's remember that the spirit of teaching encompasses partnership, acceptance, compassion, and evocation. As a trainer, you can maintain compassion for your students and empathize with their role as learners, in the same way that you once learned MI. Maintaining mindfulness of their stage of learning, learning style, and comfort participating in learning activities can help you accept the students at their current place. Partnership in learning is modeled through the type of teaching that you conduct. You also can embody the role of both facilitator of the training and participant in order to partner with your learners. Finally, use of OARS and solicitation of change talk around the behavior of using MI can allow for evocation from the learners of what they're learning and what they want to learn.

Using the spirit of MI, a trainer can respectfully and skillfully handle reservations about using MI in his or her practice—for example, using MI to address questions about how to handle "difficult patients." A common method is to preselect some of the many online videos that show examples of interactions illustrating the use of MI and those illustrating another typical encounter. The facilitator then uses the MI spirit and processes to lead a discussion of what was observed in the videos: what went well, how the patient responded, and other topics that arise.

Practice: Is This Motivational Interviewing?

Ask trainees to divide into pairs, where one is the speaker. The speaker identifies a real-life but safe change that he or she is considering but is ambivalent about ("real-play"). The partner's task is to try to convince and persuade the speaker to make the change. If resistance is encountered, the task is to persuade more emphatically. Limit the exercise to 5–10 minutes. Ask about the experience of both participants. The goal of this exercise is to elicit the experiences of both participants when persuasion, as opposed to MI, is used for behavioral change.

TEACHING THE PROCESSES OF MOTIVATIONAL INTERVIEWING

Engaging

Come to know your audience in an MI-consistent way. The positive behavior change we seek is increased competency and skillful use of MI. Use OARS to engage the learners around *their own motivation* for gaining knowledge, skills, and competence in MI. At what is the learner skillful already, and can this be used to develop competency in MI? We encourage you to remain curious about the learner.

Examples: Open Questions

"What do you already know about MI?"

"What skills do you hope to learn or practice today?"

"How can improved competence in MI help you in your work?"

Practice: Converting Questions

Have trainees practice changing closed questions into open questions. Several starting closed questions can be provided to begin the exercise, and then participants are encouraged to provide a closed question and ask another participant to make the change. Another option is to use kinesthetic signals while watching a live or video encounter. Every time a closed question is used, ask the group to put their hands together. Every time an open question is used, ask the group to open their arms wide.

Examples: Affirmations

"You're already ahead of the game on providing reflections."

"That was an excellent summary from your last MI class."

"You want to help your patients."

Practice: Affirming Strengths

Have the group of trainees identify strengths that their patients bring to treatment, and write them on a board, stated positively. Divide the strengths and trainees into equal groups, with one person assigned as an observer to report back to the larger group. Assign a set of strengths to each group and ask them to identify an open question to elicit this strength and then to provide an affirmation in response. As a class, elicit examples from each group and discuss.

Examples: Reflections

"You like the idea of MI, and you are looking for a way to feel natural when you use this with patients."

"You want MI to be more effortless in how you interact with patients who struggle to change their behaviors."

"You may not feel that MI can help solve all problems with patients, but you can see places where it might be useful."

Practice: Advancing Reflections

Have trainees divide into groups of four. One trainee reads a pre-prepared sentence stem (e.g., "I'm so sick and tired of people always telling me what to do. I mean really—where do people get off thinking they have the right to say that?"). The person to the right does a simple reflection, the next person does a paraphrased reflection, and the third person does a deep reflection (the reader reads the sentence stem three times). All trainees take turns in all roles. As a large group, discuss the experience of all participants and elicit examples of reflections done well.

Example: Summaries

"Overall, most of you here have read about MI, understand the basic processes, and have practiced some skills; but you are hoping to feel more confident in your ability to use MI and see change in your patients."

Practice: Sharing Summaries

Have trainees divide into pairs. The first person talks for 90 seconds about a real-life but safe behavior that he or she is considering changing. The other person only listens and then gives a summary of what has been said. Change the roles and repeat; but in the second set, also include a reflection of the underlying meaning, feeling, or dilemma of the story. As a large group, discuss the experience and elicit examples of reflections and summaries done well.

Focusing

Come to a shared goal for the session, informed by the process just described. Examples could include focusing on understanding the foundations of MI, collaboratively suggesting MI-consistent ways to address difficult situations the practitioners have encountered, or practicing independent role-plays with observation and feedback from peers. It can be helpful to think about how you might facilitate focusing with a patient and do this with your learners.

Practice: Focusing

Three-month priorities: Pairs of trainees work together, one as speaker and one as interviewer, to develop a list of priorities for the next 3 months. As in most of our recommended exercises, safe topics for real-play are preferred to role-play. The interviewer practices helping the speaker focus on clarifying goals and their importance, not evoking or planning. Come together as a larger group to discuss techniques used by interviewers that were helpful in focusing their priorities.

Feedback opportunity: An observer can be added to note MI-consistent behavior and share this with the group.

Agenda mapping: Have participants split into groups of two. Draw circles on a board or large piece of paper, and ask one partner to fill in some with topics for discussion as part of the training agenda (e.g., common challenges when talking to clients; how to give feedback in an MI-consistent way). Leave some empty circles, and then ask the other person to fill in these circles. Have a collaborative discussion about these topics and their significance, without choosing any particular focus yet. On the basis of the discussion, ask an open-ended question about which topic to start with first.

Evoking

Elicit change talk around MI competency and skills. Using the importance and confidence rulers (see Figures 5–2 and 5–3 in Chapter 5, "Evoking") around role-play and real-play exercises for practicing MI style and skills, one can elicit motivations for engaging in more experiential learning, then reflect or summarize that for participants.

Example

"How important, on a scale of 0 to 10, with 0 being not at all important and 10 being very important, would you say role-playing activities are for learning to use MI?" Let's say the person replies with a 4. You may then say "Okay a 4. Why not a 2?" You may get reasons such as it's safer to practice with a peer before trying with patients; the skill isn't one that can be done by simply reading; or, even though one feels put on the spot, it's a good way to get feedback.

Practice: Evoking

Drumming for change: Prepare a list of statements including preparatory and mobilizing change talk, sustain talk, and other types of statements. Read each statement aloud. Instruct trainees to remain silent if they hear sustain talk, to tap gently on their lap when they hear preparatory change talk (desire, ability, reason, need), and to drum loudly or clap their hands when they hear mobilizing change talk (commitment, activation, taking steps). Discuss any statements that have a mixed response from the audience.

Snatching change talk from the jaws of ambivalence: Prepare a list of statements that include change talk embedded within at least two pieces of sustain talk. Instruct your participants to select and then reflect the change talk, rather than do a double-sided reflection.

Dodgeball: Divide trainees into two teams. One team verbally "throws out" resistance statements or sustain talk that they have heard. The other team "dodges" resistance by responding in an MI-consistent manner (with open questions, affirmations, reflections, and summaries). Teams then switch roles. Have the larger group discuss examples that worked well.

Planning

Qualities of effective teachers include flexibility and ability to elicit ideas from the learners. In addition, many stress organization and clear objectives as important qualities. Once you have an engaged audience, a focused topic, and a sense for what motivates them to want to learn and perform MI, you can collaboratively come up with a plan for teaching using your background, knowledge, and clinical tools, combined with the needs and desires of your learners. The SMART (specific, measurable, action-oriented, realistic, time-bound) plan is helpful in thinking about planning for teaching.

Examples

"Let's practice not giving advice by completing the 'give-no-advice exercise' in the next 30 minutes as a group, and then we can come together to discuss how it went."

"We will review a video showing examples of 'reflections that go nowhere' and 'reflections that elicit more change talk' for the next 10 minutes, and then we will break into groups and practice offering reflections designed to elicit more change talk, then come together as a group to share our experiences and what worked well."

Practice: Open Questions for Planning

Trainees work in pairs to engage in a real-play exercise about something she or he would like to change. The speaker shares what she or he would like to change. The interviewer uses OARS skills to facilitate the planning with a focus on the following questions:

"What would you like to accomplish?"

"Over what period of time?"

"What steps will you take?"

"Who might help you and how?"

"What obstacles might you encounter and how will you address them?"

"How will you know you are successful?"

"Are you ready to commit to this plan?"

The trainees then switch roles.

Feedback opportunity: An observer can be added to track MI-consistent skills and mobilizing change talk.

Other Considerations

In general, learning MI should be an experiential process. Whether you are doing individual supervision or teaching a large group, finding ways for experiential learning and practice is key. You can teach MI spirit and style through role-modeling. Directing the content to development of the process instead of focusing solely on acquisition of specific skills will provide learners the ability to use and adapt MI to their specific needs and settings.

The examples provided in the practice boxes are only some of the multiple techniques available to teach MI. Please refer to www.motivationalinterviewing.org and the section "Resources" later in this chapter for a more comprehensive listing of didactic resources.

Practice: Putting It All Together With a Consult Team

Two trainees volunteer for a role-play, one to be the client and the other the interviewer, and they sit facing each other while a "consult team" sits behind the interviewer. The interviewer serves as a mouthpiece for the consult team. The client is directed to be ambivalent about making a change and has been considered by other providers to be a "difficult patient." Use this technique to go through a more thorough encounter using MI, with attention to and practice of all four processes. End the exercise with a review of what was observed and what worked well.

ENDING TRAINING

Ideally, training in MI never ends. Most experts agree on this, and most individuals who are successful in their fields (whether it be athletics, the arts, or academia) follow a similar credo. MI is a set of complex communication skills that cannot be completely imparted over a cup of coffee or simply with a single didactic experience. And very importantly, "If you don't use it, you lose it." Similar to learning a foreign language, a dance, a golf swing, to sail, or how to tie a surgical knot, the majority of learners will benefit from a combination of verbal instruction, visual modeling, and independent practice to achieve proficiency and feel confident. The level of proficiency with MI exists on a spectrum that will likely grow based on inherent ability, practice, and appropriate coaching and feedback.

MI proficiency does not always correlate with self-perception of proficiency, and a belief that the skill has been "acquired" or the "lesson learned" may decrease interest in continued training. Even health care professionals who were primed for learning (by reading a textbook) and demonstrated strong MI adherence after 2 days of training experienced tremendous skill atrophy at 4-month follow-up. At the same time, similarly motivated individuals, who underwent equivalent didactic training but received coaching or feedback intermittently after that initial didactic, maintained their skills at 4-month follow-up and continued to grow thereafter (Miller et al. 2004).

Some view the Motivational Interviewing Network of Trainers (MINT; www.motivationalinterviewing.org) as a group of individuals that perform at the pinnacle of their field and can model MI and conduct trainings. "MINTees" (and all well-intended MI practitioners) are constantly practicing, teaching, and refining their craft. Sharing this view of MI is an important component of training because it sets appropriate expectations for learners regarding goals for their initial didactic session. This view also communicates the importance of frequent practice, normalizes the need for retraining, and sets a goal toward an ideal of lifelong learning. Readers who are interested in an evaluation of their skill level or the skill level of their learners can reference the Motivational Interviewing Treatment Integrity (MITI) scale (www.motivationalinterviewing.org/content/miti-31). The scale includes instructions on its use. Viewing the scale domains can reinforce the idea that MI skills can be objectively assessed, as well as the fact that skill level may develop or atrophy with time. Helping learners appreciate that an initial, time-limited training is intended to build an essential foundation or to serve as a catalyst for a new way of interacting with their patients is a key element of setting students up for lifelong success with MI.

RESOURCES

Motivational Interviewing Practice

* Motivational Interviewing Network of Trainers: *Motivational Interviewing Training New Trainers Manual.* September 2014. Available at: http://www.motivationalinterviewing.org/sites/default/files/tnt_manual_2014_d10_20150205.pdf. Accessed December 12, 2015.

    Last updated in 2014, after the publication of the third edition of Miller and Rollnick's book on MI, this training manual is an invaluable resource containing a compilation of training ideas, exercises, and activities to incorporate during training for MI. The manual is helpfully divided into the components of MI, allowing the trainer to become familiar with a variety of activities and exercises that can be used to familiarize learners with a specific skill or concept. A variety of teaching methods are incorporated, from role-playing to writing exercises, in order to address multiple styles of learning. Importantly, as William Miller cautions in the introduction, these techniques should be tried out, practiced, and incorporated by the trainer, so as to adjust the training for one's particular style and teaching situation.

* Berg-Smith SM: *The Art of Teaching Motivational Interviewing: A Resource for MINT Trainers.* [AIM for Change Web site]. 2014. Available at: http://berg-smithtraining.com/pdf/The%20Art%20of%20Teaching%20MI%201.3.pdf. Accessed December 12, 2015.

    This manual targets MI trainers, discussing not the content that should be included in MI trainings but the process of teaching. It provides practical information about planning for and doing the training, such as preparing packets of handouts or using audiovisual aids. It also encourages trainers to develop their individual style of training, yet one that embodies the spirit of MI.

Motivational Interviewing Training

- Miller W, Yahne C, Moyers T, et al.: "A Randomized Trial of Methods to Help Clinicians Learn Motivational Interviewing." *Journal of Consulting and Clinical Psychology* 72(6):1050–1062, 2004

  In this article, Miller et al. compare outcomes among students who were exposed to four different training structures for MI. Findings include the following: Students who are primed to learn (had a baseline knowledge of MI) may gain more from MI training than individuals without baseline knowledge. Repeat exposures with bedside teaching and feedback are essential to maintaining proficiency. Teaching students to extinguish bad habits (such as confrontational language) may be as important as teaching them new skills (open questions, affirmations, reflections, summaries [OARS]) and building new habits. Additional pearls for training are scattered throughout this article. We strongly encourage that all potential trainers read the full text.

- Söderlund L, Madson M, Rubak S, et al.: "A Systematic Review of Motivational Interviewing Training for General Health Care Practitioners." *Patient Education and Counseling* 84(1):16–26, 2011

  This systematic review evaluates studies that have compared different aspects of MI training for general health care professionals. The typical duration of MI training varied from 4 hours to several days, and the common elements included in MI training were fostering MI spirit, practicing basic skills (OARS), recognizing and reinforcing change talk, rolling with resistance, and enhancing motivation. Some training sessions involved trained actors for practice of communication skills. In the other trainings, lecture attendees practiced with one another. There was no measurable benefit to including actors in the training sessions. Most studies included follow-up training. The studies that did not include follow-up training witnessed significant skill atrophy. This article may be useful to readers as they consider the content they may wish to include in a training session, and the duration of their training, and as they consider trying to structure follow-up with trainees to maintain and refine their skills after their initial training.

- Martino S, Ball S, Nich C, et al.: "Teaching Community Program Clinicians Motivational Interviewing Using Expert and Train-the-Trainer Strategies." *Addiction* 106(2):428–441, 2011

  This study evaluated the impact of different approaches to training the *leader* of MI trainings on *student* outcomes. This question was addressed by comparing student outcomes from MI trainings when the session was conducted by an expert, a leader who had undergone a structured "train the trainer" education session, or a leader who had completed a self-study protocol. An important consideration is that very few of the leaders in the self-study group actually completed the protocol as it was intended. Nonetheless, the study compares MI adherence, competence, and the percentage of students who met MI standards at baseline, postworkshop, postsupervision, and at 12-week follow-up. Students trained by an expert or by someone with a structured "train the trainer" experience had significantly higher adherence to MI strategies and communication techniques than students trained by leaders offered a self-study protocol. This study may be of interest to any person considering conducting an MI session, and it suggests that there is value in considering the training of the person conducting the MI training.

- Madson M, Loignon A, Lane C: "Training in Motivational Interviewing: A Systematic Review." *Journal of Substance Abuse Treatment* 36(1):101–109, 2009

In this article, Madson et al. reviewed 28 studies and found that the duration of training in these studies varied from a single 20-minute video to 5 weeks of training, though the majority of studies involved 9–16 hours of structured learning. Booster sessions and/or supervised bedside feedback were included in most training protocols. The authors of this review described a common eight-step progression followed by MI trainers. Most sessions begin by teaching the philosophy or spirit of MI, followed by conducting skills training in client-centered counseling, recognizing and reinforcing change talk, eliciting change talk, recognizing and rolling with resistance, developing a plan, and then helping the patient develop commitment. The final step consists of thinking about integration of MI with other strategies. This information is useful in understanding general covered topics, though there may be some differences since the third edition of the MI book by Miller and Rollnick has been published.

Lectures

- Brown G, Mangoue M: "AMEE Medical Education Guide No. 22. Refreshing Lecturing: A Guide for Lecturers." *Medical Teacher* 23(3):231–244, 2001

This article is intended as a guide for medical professionals to enhance the structure and quality of their lectures. Brown and Mangoue pay special attention to the importance of varying instructional strategies during a lecture to maintain engagement among learners. In addition to reinforcing this key concept throughout the text, the authors offer concrete tools to facilitate transitioning that concept into practice. This article is a very comprehensive resource that can be useful to both novice and senior educators.

- Hafler J: "Effective Presentations: Tips for Success." *Nature Immunology* 12(11):1021–1023, 2011

  This article is written with the understanding that "most faculty members lack knowledge of educational principles and teaching strategies, and it has been proposed that principle-based teaching competencies apply in any format of teaching." Furthermore, the author contends that faculty must complete several tasks in order to be effective, including the creation of a learning environment, use of prepared strategies to engage learners, and the development of methods for self-assessment of one's own teaching. Hafler asserts that good training in education principles improves the effectiveness of presentations. The author continues by describing the keys to developing an appropriate learning environment, how to focus a learning session, how to engage learners, and how to develop reflective skills that can lead to life-long improvement. Highlights from the text include a discussion of active learning strategies, such as discussion, group work, and brainstorming and voting; a checklist to ensure lectures will be of high quality; and, finally, practical tips regarding the importance of body language, tone, and volume to promote engagement and facilitate learning.

Large- and Small-Group Practice

- Lake F, Vickery A, Ryan G: "Teaching on the Run Tips 7: Effective Use of Questions." *Medical Journal of Australia* 182(3):126–127, 2005

  "As you question, so shall they learn" and "The more you (the teacher) talk, the less they (your students) learn" are consistent with the spirit of MI and are at the core of good pedagogy. In this article, Lake et al. offer clinicians strategies for unstructured teaching. While useful in that regard, the article can serve as an outstanding resource in structured teaching as well, because it focuses on questioning techniques. Useful strategies include incorporating the hierarchy of knowledge, providing examples of questions to determine the learner's knowledge, using questioning techniques to stimulate higher-order thinking, and describing simple skills that ensure that learners gain the most benefit from each thoughtful question their teacher poses.

- Jaques D: "Teaching Small Groups." *BMJ* 326(7387):492–494, 2003

  In this brief article, strong visual aids and clear advice help to transform a learning experience from a low-yield lecture into a high-yield, interactive educational experience. In addition to offering perspective on teaching theory, Jaques discusses practical strategies such as group rounds, buzz groups, snowball groups, fishbowls, crossover groups, and circular questioning. The strategies are useful for skill-building sessions, in which the educator is forced to repeatedly transition between large-group lecture and small-group practice. Strategies offered in this paper help learners remain engaged and offer the presenter a chance to assess skill mastery.

Providing Feedback

- Rider E, Longmaid E: "Giving Constructive Feedback." *JAMA* 274(11):876, 1995

  In this resource, Rider and Longmaid discuss concrete structure and strategies for offering feedback. These strategies can be used during bedside teaching and other informal supervision. Strategies include letting learners establish the educational goals, intentionally creating a climate of trust in which learners welcome feedback, making sure learners know they will be receiving ongoing feedback, and soliciting from learners what they did well. Recommendations include being as specific as possible and using nonjudgmental language that relates back to the learner.

KEY POINTS

- Teaching motivational interviewing (MI) is an excellent opportunity to use the spirit of MI and to model the four processes of MI as the framework for doing the training. Teaching strategies include didactic and experiential learning followed by supervision, monitoring, and feedback.

- In addition to the four processes of MI used to frame teaching, another useful framework is informed by the Gradual Release of Responsibility Model, commonly understood as the "I do it, we do it, you do it" model, that can be consistent with the MI style.

- Several activities have been developed to help trainees learn or practice the four MI processes or various MI skills and techniques that can be found in this chapter and in MI training materials available at www.motivationalinterviewing.org. There are also many video demonstrations of both MI-consistent and MI-inconsistent encounters that can illustrate many points and that are useful to vary teaching methodologies.

- Although the MI training session may end, it is helpful to think about learning MI as a perpetual process of training, skill practice, supervision, reflection, and refinement.

STUDY QUESTIONS

1. Which of the following correctly pairs the name of the component of the Gradual Release of Responsibility Model with an accurate description?

    A. "I do it." SUPERVISION/FEEDBACK. Trainees are allowed time for independent practice and making mistakes. The trainer observes (in real time or after) use of the skills, solicits trainee input about the experience, reflects trainee feedback to the trainee, affirms skills well executed, and offers summaries. The trainer can also offer observations and opportunities for improvement as appropriate.
    B. "We do it." COLLABORATION/MONITORING. The teacher participates with trainees in practicing skills, trainees practice the skill in a small group with the trainer leading the exercise, and trainees role-play among themselves, with the trainer listening and offering information and advice as appropriate.
    C. "You do it." MODELING. The teacher introduces the skill, role-models the skill, provides examples, and demonstrates use.
    D. "We do it." MODELING. The teacher introduces the skill, role-models the skill, provides examples, and demonstrates use.

2. Which of the following correctly pair a concept from the spirit of MI with an example of how to use it during MI training?

    A. *Compassion*—Approaching the learners with an attitude that MI is easy to learn if you just memorize a few mnemonic devices and that practicing it once or twice is enough to be competent.
    B. *Acceptance*—Understanding that your students have had training in how to talk to patients before and so they already know that MI can be useful to them and can see the benefit of working to develop good MI behaviors.
    C. *Partnership*—Reminding your learners that you are the expert and so copying what you do is the only way to learn MI.
    D. *Evocation*—Soliciting from learners, using open questions, their knowledge of MI and how they might find it useful.

3. Which of the following activities is a possible interactive exercise to practice focusing?

    A. *Agenda mapping:* Have participants split into groups of two. Draw circles on a board or large piece of paper, and ask one partner to fill in some with topics for discussion as part of the training agenda (e.g., common challenges when talking to clients or how to give feedback in an MI-consistent way). Leave some empty circles, and then ask the other person to fill in these circles. Have a collaborative discussion about these topics and their significance, without choosing any particular focus yet. Then, on the basis of this discussion, ask an open-ended question about which topic to start with first.

B. *Drumming for change:* Prepare a list of statements, including preparatory and mobilizing change talk, sustain talk, and other types of statements. Read each statement aloud. Instruct trainees to remain silent if they hear sustain talk, to tap gently on their lap when they hear preparatory change talk (desire, ability, reason, need), and to drum loudly or clap their hands when they hear mobilizing change talk (commitment, activation, and taking steps). Discuss any statements that have a mixed response from the audience.

C. *Snatching change talk from the jaws of ambivalence:* Prepare a list of statements that include change talk embedded within at least two pieces of sustain talk. Instruct your participants to select and then reflect the change talk, rather than do a double-sided reflection.

D. *Dodgeball:* Divide trainees into two teams. One team verbally "throws out" resistance statements or sustain talk that they have heard. The other team "dodges" resistance by responding in an MI-consistent manner (with open questions, affirmations, reflections, and summaries). Teams then switch roles. Have the larger group discuss examples that worked well.

4. Ending MI training is best done by

A. Completing a "real-play" full MI session with feedback from an observer and the opportunity to practice in both the patient and clinician roles.

B. Recording an actual MI session and then having an observer rate your use of and adherence to MI.

C. Continually training, practicing, and using MI to maintain your proficiency.

D. Recognizing when you've acquired good MI skills and continuing to use these skills similarly in all patient encounters.

5. One tool that can be used to help evaluate and objectively assess use of MI is the

A. Special Education Against Resistance in MI Network (SpEAR MINt).

B. Motivational Interviewing Treatment Integrity (MITI) scale.

C. Motivational Interviewing Group Help Training Yield scale (MIGHTY scale).

D. Motivational Interviewing National Training Team Education Assistance (MINT TEA).

REFERENCES

Frey N, Fisher D, Everlove S: Productive Group Work. How to Engage Students, Build Teamwork, and Promote Understanding. Alexandria, VA, Association for Supervision and Curriculum Development, 2009

Miller WR, Yahne CE, Moyers TB, et al: A randomized trial of methods to help clinicians learn motivational interviewing. J Consult Clin Psychol 72(6):1050–1062, 2004 15612851

STUDENT REFLECTIONS

Melissa Thomas
Yale School of Medicine, MS2

Reading this chapter as a future clinician, I realized I'll be able not only to utilize the MI skills presented in previous chapters but also to teach others to use these skills. I can see the value in training clinicians in a variety of specialties, such as those working in initial-point-of-care settings such as primary care or the emergency room who are at the potentially greatest point of impact for change in patients struggling with life modifications dealing with addiction, obesity, or diabetes, for example. Other clinicians in the mental health setting may also appreciate additional skills that are complementary to other therapy modalities as well. I particularly like the idea of helping people receive training in a skill for which they are not expected to be in an expert role and to not have the responsibility of developing the change plan or solution. Thus, teaching MI would be particularly useful in training peer mentors in the Veterans Affairs health care setting. Since peer mentors are not licensed, they are better suited for MI, which uses exploration and resolution of ambivalence rather than an expert role. Through teaching MI, I can train them to have more emphasis on acceptance and compassion, elicit what the patient understands about his or her desire to change, and focus on supporting the patient's existing strengths rather than training him or her on specific exercises. I found the "I do, we do, you do" model presented in this chapter an easy-to-follow and easy-to-understand teaching style and appreciate the examples given for how to enlist participation. Finally, I understand now that through teaching I can experience a supportive and collaborative relationship with colleagues and improve my own skills even more than could be achieved by just practice alone.

Motivational Interviewing in Administration, Management, and Leadership

Petros Levounis, M.D., M.A.

Elie G. Aoun, M.D.

> There is nothing so practical as a good theory.
>
> —*Attributed to Kurt Zadek Lewin, psychologist (1890–1947)*

Clinicians do much more than treat patients. From managing interdisciplinary teams, to directing departments and hospitals, to consulting for corporations, we are often called on to fill administrative and leadership positions. We are routinely recruited for such roles primarily because of our training in human behavior and our profound interest in what other people have to say. Although we sometimes frown on managerial tasks—"I didn't go to medical school to learn how to hold meetings!"—a number of us are finding that the principles discussed in this book apply to a wide range of activities beyond the psychotherapeutic dyad. Furthermore, managing people from a humanistic perspective can be as rewarding and gratifying as treating patients.

Whether motivating a team in the workplace to experiment with a new work schedule or planting the seed of ambivalence in an addict's mind, the path to helping people change and maintain their gains is similar. Negotiating the terms of a new contract (either of an employee or of your own) may not be all that different from convincing a patient to come to the emergency room. Ultimately, basic motivational skills such as expressing empathy and rolling with resistance can go a long way toward helping people change their behavior in many clinical and nonclinical situations.

In this chapter, we first introduce a case study of an attempt to change the culture of a health care organization. The case is explored by examining how disciplines other than behavioral sciences address motivation and change. We then apply concepts and suggestions on motivating individuals from the world of clinical service (the subject of the previous chapters of this book) to the task of changing the larger culture of a system of complex individual human beings.

THE CASE OF DNR (DO NOT READMIT) AT RECOVERY CENTRAL

To illustrate the concepts discussed in this chapter, we describe a composite and fictionalized case study.

We were asked to lead a consultation team for Recovery Central, a community mental health organization that wanted to increase its number of admissions and, consequently, improve its flailing finances. We quickly realized that the problem was not external (there were plenty of patients presenting for treatment) but internal. A number of patients were deemed by staff as untreatable or undesirable and thus were turned away. The majority of them were patients who had been treated at the facility in the past but who had relapsed. A staff member proudly told us: "We do not readmit here. What's the point? We have no interest in providing a revolving door for people who cannot take advantage of what we have to offer." And this attitude was shared widely by the rest of the staff. Our task was clear: we needed to help the organization change its culture from "just say no" to "just say yes."

We identified a number of staff misconceptions about the clinical course of substance use disorders and other mental illnesses. The idea of addiction as a chronic relapsing illness was far from familiar to the clinicians. We also made a list of other logistical barriers that had to be deconstructed and obstacles that had to be overcome so that patients could be easily admitted to the facility and receive proper care. We invited mental health experts to give in-service seminars and grand rounds lectures, mandated attendance at the training events, and made sure that everyone understood why their attitudes were outdated, uninformed, misguided, or just plain wrong. They needed to change.

We wrote tests to check the staff's knowledge, had the staff take the tests (once again, this was mandated), and put their scores in their permanent personnel files. We asked supervisors to review all cases that were deemed inappropriate for admission and incentivized the desired change by giving staff a bonus based on the number of patients admitted.

A year later, staff could recite DSM-5 diagnostic criteria for alcohol use disorder and even talk about motivational interviewing (MI). However, the number of admissions showed only modest improvement and ultimately returned to baseline. Supervisors' reviews of denied cases mostly agreed with the staff's original choices of rejecting returning patients.

The entire exercise of our consultation received high praise from everyone—they liked us! Evaluations revealed that the staff members were very impressed with our qualifications and expertise. They found us "dynamic," "visionary," and "inspirational." But change was not achieved.

WHAT WENT WRONG

Everything went wrong. Wait a minute—that's not entirely correct. We taught the staff a lot of good ideas (not unlike the ones in the book you are holding in your hands) and provided them with practical, hands-on exercises. We checked the impact of our efforts with reviews and feedback mechanisms. But it seems that we missed the mark.

Motivating people to change and maintain gains is not a task unique to the world of psychotherapy. Several endeavors share similar ambitions and, quite often, similar techniques:

- Inspiring troops in military campaigns
- Increasing industrial productivity
- Teaching and parenting
- Coaching in sports
- Leading in business
- Working the social media

In the corporate world, successfully motivating employees has become the core mission of business administration, management, and leadership. The everyday life of a basketball coach may be very different from that of a professional corporate coach, but their basic goal and process of motivating people to achieve excellence are essentially the same.

Let's review some traditional explanations of what might have happened at Recovery Central.

Military: The Art of War (circa 500 B.C.)

In *The Art of War*, one of the oldest and most popular treatises on military strategy, Sun Tzu suggests that motivating troops requires that the commander and the army be one with the Tao (Tzu 500 B.C./2003). He goes on to explain that being one with the Tao in this case means that people and their superiors work toward common goals. Although this idea seems self-evident, it is in stark contrast to the alternative strategy of the carrot and the stick, which is the bread and butter of today's approach to motivating people.

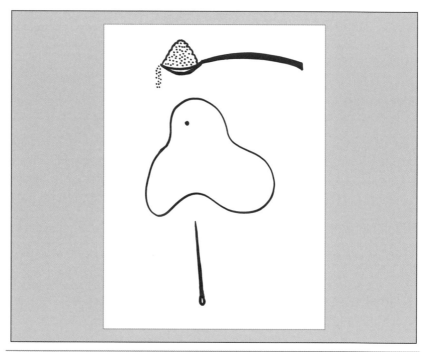

FIGURE 11–1. The amoeba theory of management.

The amoeba moves in the desired direction by being either poked with a needle or rewarded with sugar.
Source.   Adapted from Flaherty 2005. Drawing by Lukas Hassel.

James Flaherty (2005) gave another name to the carrot-and-stick tactic of motivation; he called it the "amoeba theory of management." Do you remember the amoeba experiments from high school biology labs? You could make an amoeba move in a particular direction by either poking it with a needle from the back or placing a piece of sugar in front of the protozoan (Figure 11–1). The problem here is that these techniques ignore the internal desires, fears, hopes, and goals of the amoeba itself. And people are not amoebas. Trying to motivate people by fear and punishment (needle) ultimately leads to resentment and revolution; hoping to lead by charisma and infatuation (sugar) leads to disillusionment and secrecy, as we discuss in the section "Leadership: Charisma Versus the Brutal Facts (2000s)."

Had we appreciated Sun Tzu's perspective, we might have invested more in listening than talking at Recovery Central. We clearly employed a top-down instead of bottom-up approach. Effective motivation and lasting change depend on gaining an understanding of the staff's needs and building a relationship based on common goals.

Industry: Hawthorne Effect (1920s)

In a series of studies with factory workers conducted at the Hawthorne Works manufacturing facility in Illinois between 1924 and 1932, productivity improved dramatically during the research period but returned to baseline after the investigators left the plant (Mayo 1949).

The classic interpretation of this finding is that the workers were motivated and worked harder just because they were being studied. Perhaps they feared that they were under greater scrutiny, or they responded to the experimental conditions by working as a team toward a higher goal, or they felt that they were being heard by their higher-ups. The Hawthorne effect is essentially the sociological equivalent of the well-described placebo effect in pharmacological studies.

At Recovery Central, the staff may have responded to our consultation with a combination of fear and good intentions, which resulted in the modest improvement in attitude and number of admissions. However, the positive outcomes were short-lived and returned to baseline after we concluded our consultation.

Education: What You Expect Is What You Get (1960s)

In the 1960s, Rosenthal and Jacobson (2003) expanded the ideas of the Hawthorne studies to the worlds of education and parenting. They conducted an experiment with a group of elementary school teachers as their unsuspecting subjects. At the beginning of the school year, the researchers told the teachers that some students were particularly bright; they were the "academic spurters" compared with the rest of the class. In fact, the so-called gifted students were selected randomly, and any difference between the two groups existed solely in the teachers' minds. At the end of the school year, the designated academic spurters scored considerably higher on standard IQ tests than the children who were deemed less gifted. Rosenthal and Jacobson named this self-fulfilling prophecy the "Pygmalion effect" after the mythological sculptor who fell in love with his own ivory creation.

Perhaps our expectations of the staff at Recovery Central were not high enough to effect change. More correctly, we may have hoped that they would change in the direction we wished, but we failed to allow ourselves to believe that they were truly willing (or even capable) of changing.

Sports: Self-Determination Theory (1980s)

From a sports psychology perspective, motivation for achieving athletic goals traditionally has been seen as driven by two forces: 1) external rewards and

2) internal resolve. The external force is based on operant conditioning, not unlike Flaherty's amoeba theory: people learn from the consequences of their actions and respond to environmental cues by seeking reward and avoiding punishment. The internal force was not fully appreciated until the 1984 Summer Olympics in Los Angeles, when the field of sports and exercise psychology became a scientific discipline in earnest.

The self-determination theory, formally introduced by Edward L. Deci and Richard M. Ryan in the 1980s, postulates that an athlete's behavior is primarily self-endorsed and self-determined, thus shifting the focus of motivational efforts from external to internal considerations (Deci and Ryan 1985). If the Hawthorne and Pygmalion effects point to the power of social placebos, self-determination theory reminds us that humans still maintain a degree of autonomy and free will.

At Recovery Central, the consulting team appreciated neither the cultural context of the organization nor the staff's own needs for competence and self-actualization. We steadfastly insisted on a highly directive approach, which suffocated both internal and external forces.

Leadership: Charisma Versus the Brutal Facts (2000s)

Since the 1990s, the work of Jim Collins has informed and transformed the way we think about motivation and change in the business arena (Collins 2001, 2005, 2009; Collins and Porras 1995). He boldly states that "spending time and energy trying to 'motivate' people is a waste of effort" (Collins 2001, p. 89). Helping people face brutal facts is far more helpful than giving inspirational pep talks.

On the basis of extensive research in what makes today's companies succeed or fail, Jim Collins challenges the traditional idea that a strong, charismatic, highly motivating, and visionary leader is an essential factor for positive change. In fact, charismatic leaders tend to shield others—and more importantly, be shielded from—the frequently unpleasant truth, thus becoming less effective in the long run than their less charismatic counterparts.

It is unlikely that the staff members at Recovery Central were fully forthcoming about the messy realities of their everyday work when talking with the consultation team, whose members included esteemed professors with considerable ego strengths (and, of course, egos) and personality pizzazz. Remember how we were evaluated as impressive and inspirational? Charisma might have been more of a liability than an asset for effecting lasting change.

Social Media: Ingenuity in Marketing (2010s)

Over the past decade, technological advances have revolutionized the ways humans connect and interact with one another and their cultural environment. Facebook and Instagram have replaced diaries, photo albums, and newspapers; Google has replaced the Yellow Pages; and Tinder and Grindr have provided a substitute to hanging out in social venues to meet social, romantic, and sexual partners. As a society, we have grown increasingly comfortable sharing our preferences, the highlights of our lives, and our personal thoughts and emotional states and receiving information on the Web.

Shrewd developers and data engineers have capitalized on our use of these social media venues to individualize their marketing strategies by extracting valuable personal information. Thus, it has become possible to target individuals who will be more likely to purchase a certain product or read a given news article with a particular political leaning. For example, posting pictures of your newborn child makes you more likely to receive targeted advertisements for expensive diaper brands. Similarly, following a conservative social figure makes you a target for campaigning by conservative politicians during an election year, and cruising on Grindr will get you invitations to specific gay bars and commercial products targeting gay men.

The effectiveness of social media marketing can be explained by Taylor Buckner's 1965 rumor transmission theory (Buckner 1965). Buckner asserted that the effectiveness of stating an opinion correlates with the network structure as well as the mental sets of individual actors in the network. The use of organic word of mouth, between families, friends, and neighbors (as opposed to mass media), increases the likelihood of convincing an individual that certain information is accurate or enhances his or her motivation to purchase a certain product. As such, social media can be thought of as a twenty-first-century version of word of mouth.

Relying on self-disclosures, social media marketing uses rumor transmission theory, social exchange theory (Homans 1958), and social penetration theory (Altman and Taylor 1973) to foster close relationships, which can be used to influence an individual's decision making. In effect, social networks represent a complex matrix where individualized information offers businesses the means to promote themselves.

Applying the principles described above to our consultation work at Recovery Central would have involved taking the time to get to know the individual staff members and understand what truly interested them. For example, we failed to identify people who could have taken the lead and developed expertise in resolving problems that we had identified in our initial survey. Doing so would have allowed us to capitalize on the existing talent, match resources to needs, and individualize our work to every single person rather than using a traditional one-size-fits-all approach. Engaging different staff members with distinct educational content and practice recommendations likely would have improved outcomes.

WHAT WE CAN DO

Is it possible to apply our clinical expertise in motivation and change gained from working with individual patients to changing the culture of a system? We believe so. Then how do we do it? First, we embrace the basic premise of MI that change is natural and intrinsic to humans and—by extension—to human systems.

By adopting a spirit of collaboration and expressing genuine empathy for the struggles of the people in a system that needs change, we can adapt the techniques and strategies of MI to the larger task of changing an entire cultural structure. Without repeating the treatment suggestions detailed in the previous chapters of this book (see Chapters 3 through 6), we now discuss a few motivational methods that may be particularly helpful in working with systems and organizations. We have organized this discussion according to two methodologies: 1) motivating people to change through the transtheoretical model and 2) motivating people to change through the four processes (Miller and Rollnick 2013).

Motivating People to Change Through the Transtheoretical Model

From a transtheoretical model of change (Prochaska and DiClemente 1984) perspective, our consultation at Recovery Central essentially failed primarily because we misdiagnosed the stage of change. More correctly, we did not even attempt to identify the stage of change at the organization. We behaved as though Recovery Central were fully ready for a new approach to treatment, when the reality was quite different. The system was more in the precontemplation than the preparation stage of change.

Correctly identifying the stage of change is a prerequisite for helping a system successfully navigate the precontemplation, contemplation, preparation, action, maintenance, and relapse phases of its journey.

Precontemplation

The essence of working with an organization at the precontemplation stage is planting the seed of ambivalence. Specifically, we try to identify any discrepancy between where the system is and where we would like it to be. For example, at Recovery Central the staff may have had no interest in admitting "repeat offenders" or "frequent flyers," but they still may have wanted to offer a solution to these patients' problems. Few people like to be mean, and given the opportunity, the staff would have liked to have been able to offer a mutually acceptable alternative to admission.

Another way to approach assessing a system at this stage is to ask for a description of a typical day. People invariably report both what they experience and what they wish they could experience. Capitalizing on the smallest discrepancy between reality and perfection, and eventually driving a wedge through it, is an effective way to move the system from precontemplation to contemplation.

Contemplation

At the contemplation stage of change, systems are asked to perform a cost-benefit analysis. One may use a decisional balance sheet or construct a two-by-two table: the columns identify positive and negative outcomes, whereas the rows depict what things would look like with and without the proposed changes.

Traditionally, when we try to change a system, we tend to focus on the quadrant of negative outcomes that may occur if things don't change—and sometimes the wonderful things that will happen if things do change. However, investigating all four quadrants moves the process of change more effectively.

For example, a church that is considering embracing same-sex marriages may use this framework to explore the congregation's concerns of negative publicity or divine retribution if lesbian, gay, bisexual, and transgender (LGBT) individuals start getting married at their church. Ironically, the church may get a step closer to preparation for same-sex marriages by allowing the dissenting opinions to be fully heard because such opinions will reveal little basis for the feared catastrophes associated with LGBT nuptials.

Preparation

Before appreciating the need for motivational approaches to change—and developing effective methods for evoking intrinsic motivation—helpers of all sorts tend to say, "Come see me when you are ready." Such a dismissive statement often stems less from a disinterest in helping with the task than from a lack of methodology for working with people and systems in earlier stages of change. Traditional coaches and consultants feel more competent, and thus comfortable, with the task of motivating people who are already prepared to change.

From H. A. Dorfman's (2003) *Coaching the Mental Game: Leadership Philosophies and Strategies for Peak Performance in Sports—and Everyday Life* to Max Messmer's (2011) *Motivating Employees for Dummies*, the world is full of inspirational advice—provided a person is prepared to receive it. Nonetheless, our expertise in clinical settings can still provide unique insights and recommendations in changing a culture.

In the preparation stage, motivational work focuses on developing a realistic action plan that anticipates problems and identifies solutions. However, during this time, the system is in danger of reverting to the contemplation stage of change when hit by unforeseen complications and frustrating obstacles.

For example, overwhelmed by the magnitude of the task, a country that seemed to be fully prepared to change its health care system may start rethinking the wisdom of its resolve. Ambivalence has crept back in. In this case, recruiting contemplation stage strategies may be the most effective approach.

Action

Adjusting to the new realities of the action phase can be logistically complex and emotionally taxing. Living in a new home is stressful—even if the new home is better than the old one. Cognitive-behavioral methods of identifying, avoiding, and/or coping with triggers of relapse can be very helpful both for patients and for organizations in transition. In addition, this stage may be the right time for consolidation of intrinsic motivation with extrinsic coercion.

For example, a newspaper that recently moved its entire production online may face severe demoralization of its workforce despite the accompanying financial stabilization. For journalists whose organizations are now in the black after years of being in the red, appreciating that financial well-being does not necessarily occur at the expense of quality can open the door to new ideas. Ultimately, these journalists may embrace the unique opportunities of the electronic medium instead of always longing for the "good old days" of smelling ink on paper.

Maintenance

Maintaining the gains of the changed behaviors often requires a combination of motivational, cognitive, behavioral, regulatory, disciplinary, and social approaches. After the excitement of a triumphant transformation subsides, systems have to brace for the long run.

For example, a law enforcement system that has successfully managed to change its culture and significantly reduce racial profiling from its practices may find it difficult to sustain the motivation of its members to continue fighting crime without profiling. Under stressful conditions, the old ways of thinking, feeling, and behaving feed on disappointments and frustrations, gain strength, and threaten the system with relapse.

A multifaceted program based on the following efforts lays the foundation for effective maintenance:

- An unrelenting vigilance for early signs of recurrence
- Anticipation and planning in case of relapse
- Continuous care to support self-efficacy and self-correction.

Furthermore, long-term success also calls for the system to be courageous enough to open up, go outside its strict boundaries, break walls of silence, and enable its members to engage with the larger community. For the police force in our example to sustain its cultural shift, a number of community stakeholders (sometimes disenfranchised and angry) have to be involved, heard, and genuinely understood.

Relapse

As difficult as it is not to be disappointed, it is best to accept relapse as part of the process of change. We often say that addiction is a chronic, relapsing illness, and the same principle of acceptance applies to larger systems that struggle to sustain their new identity and culture. In the subsection "Maintenance," we noted the importance of vigilance, anticipation, and preparation for relapse. When the dreaded relapse does occur, it is essential to return to and reengage in the process of change as quickly as possible.

Furthermore, identifying the elements that might have triggered the relapse and seizing the opportunities to do things differently next time may result in additional improvements and stronger stabilization of the changed culture.

For example, consider a city that has managed to nearly eliminate graffiti from its subway system by empowering its subversive citizens to engage in sports and the arts. Suddenly, as it often happens, funding for the innovative programs disappears and graffiti returns. The sooner the city council returns to the drawing board and develops alternative lower-cost programs (along with lobbying for reinstatement of funds), the higher the likelihood will be of successful re-entry to the action stage of changing the face of the city's transportation system.

Motivating People to Change Through the Four Processes

Not unlike the MI approach in clinical settings, the four core processes described in Chapters 3– 6 can be successfully applied in administrative and managerial settings. Indeed, motivating an employee to take on additional tasks in his job (or convincing a boss to give the employee a raise for that matter) is no different from helping a grandmother quit smoking after she starts using oxygen at home or an uncle quit drinking after he causes a ruckus at Thanksgiving dinner.

Active listening and thoughtful guidance through the engaging, focusing, evoking, and planning processes are essential qualities for those looking to effect change.

Engaging

The engaging phase of MI when applied to administration and management refers to fostering the business equivalent of the clinical concept of rapport building. Engaging involves collaborating on mutually negotiated and agreed-on goals as well as the tasks required to reach these goals. As such, a trusting and mutually respectful working relationship can lead to the attenuation of the power dynamic, intrinsic to any therapeutic relationship. Empowering those you are trying to motivate fosters autonomy and encourages them to take initiatives toward the desired goal. Exploring one's values, desires, goals, positivity, expectations, and hopes encourages engaging. On the other hand, quickly identifying problematic behaviors and focusing prematurely on changing them hinders engaging.

Applying the principles of engagement to large administration and management systems looking to improve their systems' operations involves the following:

- Eliciting feedback from staff, who often carry a deep understanding of the practical aspects of the execution of operations and who can provide their valuable perspective on barriers to change
- Rewarding dedication and initiative taking

Drawing staff into the process and rewarding their efforts allows for sustained and effective practical changes facilitating the leadership's goals. For example, when two hospitals merge, staff are expected to modify their behaviors to accommodate the larger operation. They are more likely to engage in the transition if they are provided with a space to share their vision for the merger, make suggestions for ways to collaborate, and express their worries and concerns. The administration can facilitate engaging by asking employees open-ended questions that invite them to bring forward their broad perspectives. Not unlike the process of engaging in clinical settings (as discussed in more detail in Chapter 3, "Engaging"), affirmations, reflections, and summaries are helpful to cement the employee's views of their administration as compassionate, trustworthy, and knowledgeable.

Focusing

In MI, focusing is the enduring process of pursuing and upholding a direction of change. It requires developing a specific agenda that delineates the goals in terms of change and adds direction to the conversation. Effecting change during the focusing phase involves a conversational rather than a prescriptive interaction, where the goals of change are negotiated rather than assumed. Such interactions help both parties feel comfortable in tolerating the uncertainty with regard to future outcomes. Focusing relies on observing the slightest clues of change talk, encouraging strengths, and pursuing openings for change. Concretely, these principles involve the following:

- Developing a clear set of mutually agreed-upon goals
- Capitalizing on and encouraging an individual's internal motivation for change
- Identifying the small yet practical steps required to reach the goals
- Maintaining a partnership in which one party can tolerate supporting how the other party wants to proceed

In helping people embrace change and come to terms with a possible ambivalence they might not feel ready to embrace, systems may use various combinations of seemingly disparate approaches:

- Directing the focus of the relationship to meet the mutually agreed-upon agenda
- Using a Rogerian (finding the common ground), nondirective, supportive approach
- Following the person's agenda and capitalizing on his or her momentum
- Following a guiding style to further the collaboration in searching for priorities

Consider, for example, the case of a Silicon Valley start-up company trying to improve productivity by encouraging their employees to work longer hours and take initiative. In order to empower their employees, the executive team meets regularly with the entire staff to explore barriers to productivity and to discuss possible solutions. They identify goals, including increasing productivity by improving quality of life and employee satisfaction. To achieve that, employees suggest various proposals to their leadership; both groups concur on catering dinner for those who stay late in the office. From an MI perspective, employees will be more likely to succeed if they are guided by defining the following:

- What they see themselves doing
- How they can use their new privileges to benefit the interest of their employers and their own careers

Evoking

With goals and direction of change identified in the focusing process, the evoking phase allows for the exploration of one's own motivation for change. As people survey the "muddy waters" of change talk, they typically allow themselves to embrace their needs, abilities, and reasons motivating change. Sustain talk also emerges in stark contrast to change talk to maintain old habits and the status quo. Indeed, the intrinsic psychological discomfort of such conflicting motivations can provide the boost to drive change. As such, ambivalence is most likely to arise during the evoking phase and frequently leads people to feel like they have reached an impasse.

We recognize that such conflict can lead to stagnation, especially when it is protracted. Change talk is facilitated by evocative open-ended questions, affirmation of one's strengths, exploration of fears that often serve to maintain sustain talk, and celebration of healthy aspirations. Specific techniques to address ambivalence include the following:

- Evoking hope and confidence
- Emphasizing past successes
- Supporting brainstorming to overcome struggles
- Eliciting commitment language

Such work leads to the development of discrepancies and resolution of ambivalence by fostering one's own motivation.

For example, a state struggling with its water conservation efforts passes new regulations requiring farmers to use more efficient, yet costly, crop-watering technology. Major agricultural corporations threaten to relocate overseas if such regulations are not reversed. These threats evoke ambivalence for the state governor and her administration. As they begin to consider succumbing to the lobbyists' demands, they review the original concerns about water shortage and its long-term consequences. In this case, ambivalence manifests as resistance, and with appropriate counsel, they consider the possible negative consequences of the proposed changes in juxtaposition with the arguments in favor of the new rule. Doing so helps the governor and her administration resolve their ambivalence toward change and renew their commitment to save water. They also remind themselves of how they struggled through a similar situation in the past (involving legislature requiring earthquake-resistant constructions) and how ultimately change prevailed with life-saving success. Instead of reversing the ordinance, the governor and her administration brainstorm to find alternative solutions, and in the end, they offer innovative incentives for people who abide by the new regulations.

Planning

Individuals can signal an augmented motivation for change and a burgeoning resolution of ambivalence by increasing the amount and intensity of change talk and exploring what it would be like to make the change. Individuals often begin taking spontaneous small steps toward change and envisioning their lives following the change. Resisting the temptation to rush through this phase and following a stepwise goal-attainment scale can be an effective framework to engage in behaviors consistent with the desired goals. Essential elements for strengthening progress through this phase include the following:

- Nonthreatening evaluation of one's progress
- Continued troubleshooting
- Recapitulation of goals and strategies
- Comfort with a resurgence of ambivalence

For example, the CEO of an advertising group introduces a new plan for dedicated customer service in order to develop stronger relationships with the company's most valuable clients. This strategy initially leads to greater business retention, yet some clients start drifting to competitors as ambivalence about the new plan creeps back in. If you listen carefully, you can hear the reappearance of doubts. "Am I paying more for a service I don't really need?" the clients ask. "Did we launch the dedicated customer service as just a gimmick?" asks the CEO. From an MI perspective, the company may need to continue evaluating, reevaluating, troubleshooting, and recapitulating its strategy at the planning phase. However, the CEO will also have lots to gain by becoming comfortable with her clients', as well as her own, resurging ambivalence.

Finally, we would like to offer a word of caution. One of the greatest challenges for both clinical and nonclinical motivational work is limiting the ambition of the helper. People who hold advice-dispensing positions tend to be quite efficient and effective in achieving goals in their own lives and thus expect immediate change in others. More often than not, simply identifying the problem, helping an individual or culture move a little forward, supporting them at their new phase, and following up is enough. Faster, more ambitious timetables run the risk of overreaching. Ultimately, a humanistic approach that focuses on communication, collaboration, and the intrinsic motivation of people to change is often the key to success.

KEY POINTS

- Motivational interviewing (MI) concepts, developed to facilitate change in individuals, can be applied to changing the culture of systems composed of individuals.

- When using the transtheoretical model, apply the following:
  1. In the precontemplation stage, plant the seed of ambivalence.
  2. In the contemplation stage, explore both the positive and the negative prospects of life with and without the proposed change in culture.
  3. In the preparation stage, develop a realistic action plan that anticipates problems and identifies solutions.
  4. During the action stage, consolidate intrinsic motivation with extrinsic coercion.
  5. In the maintenance stage, use a multitude of motivational and psychosocial approaches to sustain the desired change.
  6. If relapse occurs, accept it as an opportunity to reengage, rethink, and reemerge stronger than before.

- When using the four-processes model, implement the following:
  1. Engage people on mutually negotiated and agreed-upon goals and potentially the tasks required to reach these goals.
  2. Focus on pursuing and upholding a direction of change, while tolerating the uncertainty intrinsic to change.
  3. Evoke change talk and manage sustain talk. Develop discrepancies, foster motivation, and resolve ambivalence.
  4. Plan for the long run by setting up achievable, yet gradually challenging, goals.
  5. Throughout the process, celebrate communication, collaboration, and the intrinsic motivation of individuals.

STUDY QUESTIONS

1. A Greek family rethinks its cooking strategies. On one hand, the health benefits of a lower-fat diet are well understood and appreciated. On the other, *fasolakia ladera* are not really *ladera* unless they happily swim in a sea of olive oil. Ambivalence and tension reign in the family. What's the stage of change?

    A. Precontemplation.
    B. Contemplation.
    C. Preparation.
    D. Action.

2. After weeks of back-and-forth, your boss says: "I am trying to think of ways I can approve your salary increase by 20% as you are asking. One option is to expect more work from you, but I worry that my chief financial officer will not be too happy with the decision." What MI process does this case exemplify?

    A. Engaging.
    B. Focusing.
    C. Evoking.
    D. Planning.

3. Three friends are stranded in an elevator without their cell phones. One of them keeps buzzing the alarm bell and screams for help while another looks for a way out. The third friend waits for the other two to figure it out. This is an example of the

    A. Hawthorne effect.
    B. Pygmalion effect.
    C. Self-determination theory.
    D. Rumor transmission theory.

4. According to Jim Collins's analysis of successful companies, a leader's charisma is

    A. More likely to be a liability than an asset.
    B. More likely to be an asset than a liability.
    C. Irrelevant to success or failure.
    D. More important than the facts in motivating people.

5. After having spent several months trying to convince your graphic designer to take 3-D courses in order to improve the quality of your products, he finally agrees. Two days later, he comes back and tells you that he changed his mind. Which of the following strategies will be most helpful in motivating him?

    A. Affirming one's strengths.
    B. Continued troubleshooting and recapitulation of goals.
    C. Following a guiding style.
    D. Developing discrepancies and resolving ambivalence.

REFERENCES

Altman I, Taylor DA: Social Penetration: The Development of Interpersonal Relationships. New York, Holt, Rinehart & Winston, 1973

Buckner T: A theory of rumor transmission. Public Opinion Quarterly. 65(29):1, 54–70, 1965

Collins J: Good to Great: Why Some Companies Make the Leap…and Others Don't. New York, HarperCollins, 2001

Collins J: Good to Great and the Social Sectors: A Monograph to Accompany Good to Great. Boulder, CO, Jim Collins, 2005

Collins J: How the Mighty Fall: And Why Some Companies Never Give In. Boulder, CO, Jim Collins, 2009

Collins J, Porras JI: Built to Last: Successful Habits of Visionary Companies. New York, HarperCollins, 1995

Deci EL, Ryan RM: Intrinsic Motivation and Self-Determination in Human Behavior. New York, Plenum, 1985

Dorfman HA: Coaching the Mental Game: Leadership Philosophies and Strategies for Peak Performance in Sports—and Everyday Life. Lanham, MD, Taylor Trade Publishing, 2003

Flaherty J: Coaching: Evoking Excellence in Others. Oxford, UK, Elsevier, 2005

Homans GC: Social behavior as exchange. Am J Sociol 63:597–606, 1958

Mayo E: Hawthorne and the Western Electric Company, The Social Problems of an Industrial Civilization. London, Routledge, 1949

Messmer M: Motivating Employees for Dummies. New York, Wiley, 2011

Miller WR, Rollnick S: Motivational Interviewing: Helping People Change, 3rd Edition. New York, Guilford, 2013

Prochaska JO, DiClemente CC: The Transtheoretical Approach: Crossing Traditional Boundaries of Therapy. Homewood, IL, Dow Jones-Irwin, 1984

Rosenthal R, Jacobson L: Pygmalion in the Classroom: Teacher Expectation and Pupils' Intellectual Development. Norwalk, CT, Crown House, 2003

Tzu S: The Art of War (circa 500 B.C.). Translated by Lionel Giles and edited by Dallas Galvin. New York, Barnes and Noble Classics, 2003

STUDENT REFLECTIONS

Jose Medina, M.S.W.
Rutgers New Jersey Medical School, MS-II

Medical school is more than the collection of coursework, clerkships, and away rotations that we progress through over our 4 years of training. As students we lead campus organizations, research projects, community service events, and more. The success of these endeavors, much like those described in this chapter, relies on the cohesiveness, relationships, and common goal setting forged by all of those involved. As a student leader on my own campus, although well intentioned, I've found that many of my own projects have fallen short of meeting expectations.

Much as this chapter uses the example of Recovery Central to paint the pitfalls of an attempt to motivate change throughout a large health system, I was able to analyze previous projects and attempts to motivate groups of volunteers through the use of the four-processes model. Through this exercise, I was able to come to terms with missteps in leadership I've made along the way. More importantly, however, in reading this chapter and putting to use the outlines provided to motivate people and systems to change, I've been able to start off on the right foot in engaging fellow student leaders and organization members as we plan for the start of the new semester. Through conversation, and dedication of time and effort in getting to know the goals, expectations, and hopes of all group members, there is unprecedented buy-in and initiative taking than ever before.

I foresee that throughout the later stages of my medical career, placing importance on communication and relationship building, and learning the internal motivators that drive the individuals on the team around me, will most certainly be the key to the entire team's having a greater chance of being successful in accomplishing the goals that we have mutually set.

The Science of Motivational Interviewing

Michelle C. Acosta, Ph.D.
Angela R. Bethea-Walsh, Ph.D.
Deborah L. Haller, Ph.D.

Motivational interviewing (MI) is one type of psychotherapy; it has been particularly well studied. In this chapter, we will 1) review the research focusing on MI, including if and how it works; 2) recommend steps toward becoming a competent MI clinician and/or researcher; 3) review how outcomes are measured to assess change when using MI; and 4) discuss implementing MI in treatment settings based on research findings.

There is an increased need for clinicians to provide evidence-based treatments. But what are evidence-based treatments, and how do they differ from standard care? Evidence-based treatments are those that have been studied scientifically and have been found to be effective in controlled studies. Controlled studies are ones in which near-optimal results might be expected because all clinicians are well trained, follow a treatment protocol, and are closely supervised. The effectiveness of the treatment compared with standard treatment (or with another evidence-based treatment) is determined by assessing the extent to which predetermined outcomes are met for patients treated using each approach. When patient outcomes are better for those receiving the experimental treatment, we say that this treatment has promise or efficacy. When the outcomes for the experimental treatment are comparable to those attained by other approaches, we are able to show that the experimental treatment is as good as approaches already in use (standard care).

By using evidence-based treatment, we are providing patients with treatment that has the best chance of working. In addition, third-party payers often require providers to employ evidence-based treatments and to measure clinical change in objective ways. Furthermore, many clinicians can use feedback about their own performance to improve their skills and their ability to help their patients. Finally, program managers and administrators want to know which treatment approaches are most likely to achieve the best outcomes in the shortest period of time and at the lowest cost. Information provided from scientific research can help to answer these questions and to improve patient outcomes, therapist skills, and program development.

How Do I Know What Motivational Interviewing Is (and Isn't)?

MI is a person-centered intervention that focuses on enhancing one's motivation in order to change a negative behavior or promote a positive behavior (Miller and Rollnick 2013). This process is thought to occur through a combination of eliciting of an individual's arguments for positive change and developing an empathic relationship in order to best support this positive change (Miller and Rose 2009). Like dynamic approaches, MI recognizes the importance of ambivalence to change; unlike dynamic approaches, MI does not employ confrontation, interpretation, or a focus on the past to resolve the ambivalence. MI uses a supportive, patient-centered, hopeful approach, yet differs from supportive therapy in that it is strategic and goal oriented. Compared with cognitive-behavioral therapy (CBT), MI places more emphasis on acceptance and compassion and less on specific exercises and strategies. For example, MI strives to evoke solutions from the patient, as opposed to instructing the patient in ways to solve his or her problems.

Both traditional drug counseling and MI employ feedback; however, the tone tends to be different. Whereas patients in drug counseling may be confronted about positive drug tests, those in MI would be encouraged to view such results as a sign of reluctance to change their drug use behavior. In addition, drug counseling tends to be pathology based, labeling patients as mentally ill, personality disordered, or addicts. In contrast, MI avoids labeling to focus more on supporting existing strengths. Drug counseling and MI do have some elements in common, including being goal directive and attempting to identify barriers to change and ways to overcome these.

Table 12–1 compares and contrasts elements of MI with other common treatment approaches. MI is most commonly used as a stand-alone treatment (only MI is provided); as an adjunctive treatment (either preceding or occurring in parallel with other medical or psychosocial treatment, usually to promote treat-

TABLE 12–1. Comparing elements of motivational interviewing (MI) with other treatment approaches

Therapeutic construct	MI	Dynamic	Supportive	CBT	Traditional drug counseling
Person centered	✓	✓			
Reflective	✓	✓			
Nonjudgmental	✓		✓		
Focus on ambivalence	✓	✓			
Solution oriented	✓				
Strategic	✓			✓	✓
Confrontational		✓		✓	✓
Focus on interpretation		✓			
Instructive/ directive				✓	✓
Focus on skills building				✓	

Note. CBT=cognitive-behavioral therapy.

ment engagement or adherence); or as a blended intervention, in which MI is combined with other therapeutic strategies into a single intervention. Many published studies involve adaptations of MI (or blended MI interventions). However, we have restricted Table 12–1 to studies of stand-alone MI for clarity.

It may also be helpful to review briefly how the definition of MI has evolved since the original publication of this chapter (Acosta et al. 2010) and the original MI textbook. One of the major changes is how MI considers the concept of resistance. Miller and Rollnick (2013) have redefined "resistance to change" both as a patient's commitment to sustain the current behavior (e.g., sustain talk) and as relationship discord. This places responsibility on the therapist to elicit patient motivation and enhance rapport. In addition to this change, Miller and Rollnick (2013) have expanded MI spirit to include acceptance and compassion as key elements, along with a collaborative, evoking spirit that promotes patient autonomy. Finally, the original four principles of MI (express empathy, develop discrepancy, roll with resistance, and support self-efficacy) have been redefined as four processes: engaging, focusing, evoking, and planning (Miller and Rollnick 2013). These refinements in MI have been informed clinically, and through emerging research that is attempting to identify the mechanisms through which MI and MI interventions promote positive change.

DOES MOTIVATIONAL INTERVIEWING WORK?

MI has been studied extensively and has been shown to be efficacious for varied problems and across different patient populations. Hundreds of studies and dozens of meta-analyses and literature reviews (i.e., papers that synthesize findings from multiple published studies) have reported that MI and MI adaptations are effective in reducing substance use (i.e., tobacco, alcohol, drugs), HIV risk, and gambling and in improving behavioral and psychiatric health, including intervention adherence and retention, diet and exercise, chronic disease management (e.g., hypertension, diabetes), and psychiatric symptoms (Dunn et al. 2001; Jones et al. 2014; Lundahl and Burke 2009; Lundahl et al. 2010, 2013; Madson et al. 2016; Rubak et al. 2005). In addition, recent studies demonstrate that MI can improve nonspecific therapeutic factors such as engagement in treatment, intention to change the problem behavior, and self-reported psychiatric distress among adults (e.g., Lundahl et al. 2010). Furthermore, MI's effects appear to last for several months after ending treatment and possibly as long as 2 years, although more research on the durability of MI is needed (Lundahl et al. 2010).

More recent research has begun to examine MI interventions for an increasingly broad range of patient populations. MI interventions have begun to show promise in reducing substance use and improving behavior health and treatment engagement among adolescents, persons involved in criminal justice settings, persons with eating disorders, and different medical populations. MI interventions have shown good acceptability and efficacy in reducing adolescent substance use and improving health behaviors (e.g., sexual risk behavior, physical activity, diet) (Cushing et al. 2014; Jensen et al. 2011). However, it may be important to consider moderating factors in treatment, because one study found that having depression reduced the effectiveness of MI for adolescents (Clair-Michaud et al. 2016). Another setting in which MI interventions are being actively tested is the criminal justice setting. Generally, studies have shown positive results for MI interventions in engaging offenders and probationers in treatment, but findings are less clear for reducing substance use (McMurran 2009). In addition, a systematic review found strong support for MI's effectiveness in managing lifestyle and psychosocial issues among cancer patients, but more modest effects were found for disease self-management (Spencer and Wheeler 2016). Research also indicates that MI may be effective in increasing motivation to change and treatment engagement in other medical populations, such as persons with chronic pain (Alperstein and Sharpe 2016) and persons with eating disorders (Macdonald et al. 2012).

Although evidence is broadly supportive of MI's effectiveness in these areas, findings continue to be mixed. For example, evidence for MI's effectiveness in improving oral health is currently mixed, although the work in these areas is generally newer (Cascaes et al. 2014; Gao et al. 2014). In a review of four meta-analyses, Lundahl and Burke (2009) reported that MI showed the strongest evidence of efficacy when compared with "weak" comparison groups, like standard care or wait-list control groups, as opposed to "strong" comparison groups, like other effective treatments, although MI did appear to have similar effects over a shorter duration compared with other effective treatments. In general, the effect size, or strength, of MI is small to moderate across different studies and may vary according to patient characteristics, the behavior or symptom being targeted by the intervention, or the format in which the intervention is delivered (Lundahl and Burke 2009; Lundahl et al. 2010, 2013; Madson et al. 2016). For example, findings are mixed when examining the effectiveness of MI interventions for ethnic and racial minority populations, with MI being more effective in minority populations (Hettema et al. 2005; Lundahl et al. 2010).

In addition to patient characteristics, studies indicate that the format in which MI is delivered may impact its efficacy. A meta-analysis found that stand-alone MI may be most effective as a brief lead-in to treatment (i.e., to increase engagement in subsequent medical or other behavioral treatment), whereas a popular MI adaptation, motivational enhancement therapy, can be an effective intervention on its own (Lundahl and Burke 2009). In addition, MI is frequently used as a single-session intervention as part of a screening, brief intervention, and referral to treatment (SBIRT) approach in health care settings (Substance Abuse and Mental Health Services Administration 2013). These brief MI interventions have shown positive outcomes for reducing smoking and hazardous drinking (Dunn et al. 2001; Vasilaki et al. 2006), but findings are less robust when risky drug use is the target (Marsden et al. 2006; Saitz et al. 2014). Finally, MI delivered in group formats may be less potent than MI delivered in one-on-one contexts, although studies examining the efficacy of group MI show mixed results (D'Amico et al. 2013; Hustad et al. 2014; Lundahl and Burke 2009).

One issue that complicates the question of whether or not MI works has been a lack of rigor regarding its implementation in MI treatment studies. Specifically, many studies have failed to provide information on treatment fidelity or the process through which one is assured that the intervention is being conducted as intended (e.g., that the MI delivered was faithful to the description provided by Miller and Rollnick [2013]). Therefore, it is possible that some studies may have reported that MI did not work, when, in fact, the clinicians were not actually providing MI. One study found that the patients of clinicians who showed higher levels of empathy and MI spirit showed significantly better outcomes than the patients of clinicians whose approach was assessed as having lower fidelity to MI spirit (Spohr et al. 2016). This issue begs the question of how MI works: what are the essential "ingredients" of MI that may promote positive change? While this question has not yet been definitively answered, we review what is known about the "how" of MI in the section "How Does Motivational Interviewing Work?"

In sum, the research literature generally supports MI and its adaptations as effective treatments for a wide and increasing variety of problem behaviors and populations. MI and one of its common adaptations, motivational enhancement therapy, have been listed as evidence-based practices in two prominent compendia of evidence-based treatments for substance use disorders: the National Registry of Evidence-based Programs and Practices (sponsored by the U.S. Department of Health and Human Services, Substance Abuse and Mental Health Services Administration), as part of their legacy programs, and the National Quality Forum (sponsored by the U.S. Department of Health and Human Services, Centers for Medicare and Medicaid Services, and the Assistant Secretary for Planning and Evaluation). How MI works and what aspects of MI are necessary to promote change are questions that have prompted a burgeoning field of research.

How Does Motivational Interviewing Work?

For all treatments, identifying the mechanisms of action, or elements necessary for the treatment to work, is important in refining the treatment and training clinicians how to effectively administer treatment. There has been a significant, recent increase in the research pertaining to understanding how MI promotes positive change and what the mechanisms for change are within MI. Most prior work focused on identifying and characterizing the essential ingredients of MI—specifically the therapist and patient processes that have been theorized as necessary to promote positive change, based on the Miller and Rollnick (1991, 2013) descriptions of MI. Most recently, it has been theorized that there are two essential, parallel processes in MI—the MI spirit that forges a supportive and collaborative environment and the four MI-specific processes of engaging, focusing, evoking, and planning that promote change when the patient is ready (Miller and Rollnick 2013).

There is good evidence to suggest that the MI spirit acts as an important mechanism of change. A systematic review was done on 37 studies dating back to 1980, including more than 5,000 participants (Copeland et al. 2015). Potential mechanisms of change examined included therapist behaviors (i.e., empathy,

MI spirit, open questions, reflections, MI-consistent behaviors, MI-inconsistent behaviors) and patient behaviors (i.e., change talk, sustain talk, self-efficacy, self-monitoring, stage of change, motivation, planning, therapeutic alliance, commitment strength, perceived control). With respect to therapist behaviors, while all therapist behaviors had some support (at least one study showed a significant mediating effect of the therapist behavior being examined), the most robust predictor of positive outcomes was MI spirit. In sum, clinicians who demonstrated higher levels of MI spirit had patients who did significantly better on a range of outcomes. Similarly, while all patient behaviors had some support, patient motivation was the strongest predictor of change within the MI treatment context. Interestingly, while self-efficacy for change was one of the most widely studied potential mechanisms for change, there was little support indicating that it serves as a mechanism for change (Copeland et al. 2015). A second meta-analysis including 19 studies (Apodaca and Longabaugh 2009) also examined therapist behaviors (e.g., MI spirit, MI-consistent behaviors, MI-inconsistent behaviors, use of specific techniques) and patient behaviors (i.e., change talk/intention, readiness to change, involvement/engagement, resistance, experience of discrepancy) as potential mediators. Apodaca and Longabaugh (2009) identified lower levels of therapist MI-inconsistent behavior and higher levels of patient change talk/intention and experience of discrepancy as the most consistent predictors of positive change.

Regarding the specific processes of MI, a growing body of research has focused on a clinician's ability to evoke patient change talk as a potential mechanism of change. Research has now demonstrated that clinician behavior can evoke change talk in patients (Glynn and Moyers 2010). A meta-analysis of studies examined the influence of therapist behavior on change and sustain talk within MI interventions. The researchers showed that therapist MI-consistent behaviors yielded higher rates of change talk in patients, while MI-inconsistent behaviors yielded lower rates of change talk and higher rates of sustain talk (Morgenstern et al. 2012). However, the relationship may be more complex, because one study demonstrated a bidirectional relationship between clinician and patient language within sessions. Specifically, clinicians were able to evoke patient change talk with positive reflections, and patients were able to elicit positive reflections from clinicians with change talk and negative reflections with sustain talk (Barnett et al. 2014). While earlier studies found support that patient change talk is related to positive outcomes (e.g., Amrhein et al. 2003; Moyers et al. 2007; Strang and McCambridge 2004), a recent meta-analysis found that the impact of change talk on outcomes was inconsistent (Morgenstern et al. 2012). Work in this area is ongoing and may help to inform further refinement of MI's core processes in future iterations.

In sum, while the literature on how MI works is a complex and growing area of research, some consistent findings have emerged. Therapist MI spirit appears to be related to better treatment engagement and outcomes across a variety of problem behaviors and patient groups. In addition, patient motivation and change talk have emerged as potential mechanisms of positive change. A clinician's ability to evoke change and sustain talk is another potential change agent, although findings are less robust. There is a need for continued work in this area and a more nuanced examination of how potential mechanisms of change may interact with each other to promote positive change. For example, Miller and Rose (2015) found that the ability of certain MI-consistent strategies to promote positive change is dependent on a patient's readiness to change.

How Do I Learn Motivational Interviewing?

There is compelling evidence that people from a wide variety of backgrounds can learn MI, including health and mental health care professionals (e.g., nurses, dieticians, counselors, social workers), clergy, and laypeople, including peers (Lundahl et al. 2010; Madson et al. 2009; Söderlund et al. 2011). However, while there is evidence that people of varied training and backgrounds can learn MI, there is evidence that some individuals and some groups of clinicians are able to learn MI more easily than others. For example, in a study of MI trainings for mental health clinicians, substance abuse clinicians, general health providers, and corrections staff, mental health clinicians showed the fewest and corrections staff the most MI-inconsistent behaviors during the training (Schumacher et al. 2014). In addition, individuals who exhibit higher levels of empathy may learn MI more easily than those who exhibit lower levels of empathy (e.g., Wolfe et al. 2013).

Miller and Moyers (2006) have outlined several stages describing what people do during MI training, with the initial stages focusing on having clinicians learn about the philosophy and spirit of MI and the later stages focusing more on the essential processes of MI, particularly evoking change talk. Typical MI training begins with a workshop, often lasting 2 days, conducted by an expert in MI (Madson et al. 2009). There is a network of clinicians, called Motivational Interviewing Network of Trainers, who have demonstrated MI proficiency and who are educated in the training and supervision of MI. Training typically includes didactics, experiential exercises, and real play (i.e., a dyad with a helper and speaker wherein the speaker discusses a topic they feel safe sharing and about which they actually feel ambivalent). While there is research that demonstrates that a single MI workshop can significantly improve MI spirit among a group of clinicians (e.g., Brug et al. 2007), other research has indicated that it is not sufficient for clinicians to become proficient in MI (Miller and Mount 2001). However, clinicians who receive continued supervision via telephone and/or feedback on audiotaped practice sessions are able to achieve mastery

(Miller et al. 2004). A meta-analysis of training studies was conducted, and this analysis demonstrated that MI workshops did produce significant gains in clinicians' MI skills across studies. However, MI skills were only sustained with an average of three to four postworkshop feedback and coaching sessions (Schwalbe et al. 2014). This suggests that while attending a workshop might be a good starting place, in order to truly learn MI many clinicians may require ongoing supervision from someone with MI mastery.

HOW DO I KNOW I'M DOING IT RIGHT?

One of the ways in which clinical research differs from standard care is the extent to which the clinician is evaluated. In standard care, clinicians either monitor themselves or are evaluated by supervisors, usually by providing supervisors a brief account of the intervention and patient progress. In contrast, most research studies use other people, including supervisors and outside raters, to evaluate clinician performance. Supervision in research studies is often audiotaped or videotaped, and feedback is provided to the clinician. In contrast, outside raters listen to or watch session tapes and complete rating measures, although typically they do not provide feedback directly to study clinicians. The reason clinicians are evaluated so much more thoroughly in research studies is to ensure treatment fidelity. Treatment fidelity has to do with how well clinicians can learn the intervention and how accurately they can deliver the intervention according to the treatment manual, study protocol, or theoretical approach (see Table 12–3 later in this chapter). Treatment fidelity is important in clinical research for a variety of reasons. First, if clinicians are unable to learn the intervention, it suggests that the intervention is not feasible. Second, if clinicians do not deliver the intervention appropriately, it will be impossible to know if patient outcomes are a function of the intervention or are due to other factors. In addition, if clinicians are unable to perform the intervention in a standardized way (i.e., all clinicians carry out the intervention in the same way), then other researchers and clinicians will not be able to replicate the results of the study.

　　The first step to ensure treatment fidelity is training the clinicians. As stated in the section "How Do I Learn Motivational Interviewing?" initial training typically consists of a workshop. After training, clinician skills are evaluated, and often the clinicians are given "pilot" or "test" patients and monitored closely to make sure that they are performing the intervention as directed. Once they achieve mastery, clinicians are allowed to begin delivering the intervention with ongoing supervision. Clinicians are supervised and rated via audiotape or videotape or in-person observation. Raters use a standardized measure to evaluate clinician tapes or observed sessions. There are many tools available for raters to use (Table 12–2), and the tools vary in length and content. Raters are typically well trained in MI and have a good working knowledge of the intervention. Most measures of fidelity require the rater to review the tape and then evaluate the clinician on a number of items. In addition, some measures require that the clinician keep a behavioral tally of specific clinician behaviors in session.

The rating scales presented in Table 12–2 are general MI style tools. However, rating scales may be adapted to incorporate different items from the intervention, using the manual as a guide. Clinicians also may use the intervention manual or other standardized intervention materials to assist in intervention delivery. Although most studies provide manuals to assist in training and ensure fidelity, a meta-analysis of MI studies indicated that studies that did not use a manual for MI yielded better patient outcomes (Hettema et al. 2005). Unfortunately, many clinicians have difficulties learning an intervention without a manual or guide, especially if the intervention incorporates other strategies (e.g., CBT) in addition to MI.

Manuals and periodic retraining also are useful in preventing *drift*, which is when clinicians drift back to their own style and away from the intervention. In addition to ensuring that clinicians remain well trained and adherent to the intervention, researchers also are concerned with something called *contamination*. Contamination occurs when a clinician is exposed to, and incorporates, elements of another intervention condition into his or her intervention delivery. Researchers try to prevent this from occurring in multiple ways, including having clinicians deliver different interventions at separate sites. In addition to close monitoring of the clinicians, patients/participants are often asked or given measures to assess their perceptions of the intervention and/or the clinician.

HOW DO I KNOW WHEN MOTIVATIONAL INTERVIEWING IS WORKING FOR MY PATIENTS? (ARE MY PATIENTS CHANGING?)

Like most interventions, there are several ways to see whether or not MI is working, both for individual patients and for groups of patients. One of the most common ways researchers and clinicians determine whether or not an intervention is working is to track specific patient goal-oriented outcomes. In standard care, individual goal-oriented outcomes are those outcomes that patients hope to change or improve. For example, a patient may want to reduce his or her depressive symptoms or may want to reduce drug use. Individual goal-oriented outcomes are often tracked regularly on treatment plans or through the regular use of objective assessments, including clinical instruments like the Beck Depression Inventory (Beck et al. 1996) or urine toxicology screens. If patients show change in their goal-oriented outcomes (e.g., lower scores on the Beck Depres-

TABLE 12–2. Tools to assess treatment engagement, change process, and satisfaction with treatment

Scale	What it consists of	What it measures
Working Alliance Inventory (Horvath and Greenberg 1989)	36 items rated on a 7-point Likert scale Therapist, client, and observer versions	Scores for agreement on tasks, agreement on goals, and strength of bond between therapist and client
The Working Alliance Inventory— Short Form Revised (Hatcher and Gillaspy 2006)	12 items rated on a 5-point Likert scale Therapist and client versions	Scores for agreement on tasks, agreement on goals, and strength of bond between therapist and client
Helping Alliance Questionnaire–II (Luborsky et al. 1996)	19 items rated on a 6-point Likert scale Therapist and client versions	Score for overall helping alliance
California Psychotherapy Alliance Scale (Gaston and Marmar 1994)	24 items rated on a 7-point Likert scale Therapist and client versions	Scores for overall therapeutic alliance and four scales: Patient Working Capacity, Patient Commitment, Therapist Understanding and Involvement, and Working Strategy Consensus
URICA (Blanchard et al. 2003; McConnaughy et al. 1982)	32 items rated on a 5-point Likert scale	Score on each of four stages of change: precontemplation, contemplation, action, and maintenance; also scores on readiness to change and commitment to action
Stages of Change Algorithm (Velicer et al. 1995)	3–5 stepped questions	Places person within a single stage of change: precontemplation, contemplation, preparation, action, and maintenance

TABLE 12–2.   Tools to assess treatment engagement, change process, and satisfaction with treatment *(continued)*

Scale	What it consists of	What it measures
SOCRATES (Miller and Tonigan 1996)	19-items rated on a 5-point Likert scale	Scores for ambivalence, recognition, and taking steps
Decisional Balance Scale (Velicer et al. 1985)	10–20 items depending on change behavior, rated on 5-point Likert scale	Scores for pros of change and cons of change
Treatment Motivation Scale (Knight et al. 1994)	29 items rated on a 5- or 7-point Likert scale	Scores for overall treatment readiness
Client Satisfaction Questionnaire (Larsen et al. 1979)	8 items rated on a 4-point Likert scale	Score for overall satisfaction with treatment

Note.   SOCRATES = Stages of Change Readiness and Treatment Eagerness Scale; URICA = University of Rhode Island Change Assessment.

sion Inventory), then one might infer that the intervention is working. However, it is difficult to determine the extent to which an intervention is working for the individual and the extent to which external factors may be influencing outcomes. One way to feel more confident that the intervention is the active agent of change is to examine change in a group of patients or to compare two groups of patients receiving different interventions. Group outcomes may be tracked by collapsing individual goal-oriented outcomes. For example, in an alcohol treatment program, one might track days abstinent from alcohol across all patients. However, this approach is sometimes difficult in more general standard care settings, because individual patients often have different goal-oriented outcomes.

In addition to goal-oriented outcomes, patients may exhibit change in process outcomes. Process outcomes include patient attendance/retention in treatment, therapeutic alliance, or satisfaction with services. In addition to these general process outcomes, there are process outcomes specific to MI, including motivation to change and stage of change. Stages of change include precontemplation, contemplation, preparation, action, and maintenance (Prochaska and DiClemente 1983). *Precontemplation* is when patients either do not believe they have a problem or recognize the problem but do not want to change. *Contemplation* is when patients begin to think about changing their problematic behaviors, and *preparation* is when patients begin to plan out or to take their first steps toward change. *Action* is when patients begin to fully engage in behavior change, whereas *maintenance* occurs when the behavior change has been sustained for some period of time. Patients may enter treatment in one of the early stages of change (e.g., precontemplation, contemplation), and one way to evaluate an intervention is to determine whether or not patients are moving through the stages of change. For individual patients, one may compare their stage of change at the beginning of treatment with their stage of change at various subsequent follow-up time points (e.g., every 3 months, halfway through treatment, at the end of treatment). When examining groups of patients, one may want to compare the percentage of patients at different stages of changes at the beginning of treatment with the percentage of patients at subsequent time points. Another way to measure the change process is to measure the more general concept of readiness or motivation to change. Readiness to change is a way of thinking about all of the stages in a fluid way; patients in the precontemplation stage are lowest and patients in the maintenance stage are highest on a readiness to change continuum. Standardized measures to assess the change process can be found in Table 12–3. Most are fairly short and are easy to administer and score.

In-session progress can also be examined for individuals and for groups, although this is often a much more time-consuming and difficult task. In-session progress may be assessed by looking at the language that patients use in session because there is early evidence that patient language is a good indicator of behavior change (Amrhein et al. 2003; Apodaca and Longabaugh 2009; Moyers

TABLE 12–3. Tools to assess adherence and competence while implementing motivational interviewing (MI) intervention

Scale	What it consists of	What it measures
Motivational Interviewing Treatment Integrity (MITI) Coding Manual 4.2.1[a]	A behavioral coding system with two components: global scores on a 5-point Likert scale and behavior counts of therapist behaviors	Global scores across four dimensions (cultivating change talk, softening sustain talk, partnership, and empathy); behavior tallies (questions, persuasion, reflections, MI-adherent behaviors, MI-nonadherent behaviors)
Motivational Interviewing Skills Code (MISC; Moyers et al. 2003)	Three views of the audiotape/videotape for three different scales using a 7-point Likert scale after each review	Three ratings: Global Therapist Rating (acceptance, egalitarianism, empathy, genuineness, warmth, and spirit of MI), Global Patient Rating (affect, cooperation, disclosure, and engagement), and the Global Interaction Rating (level of collaboration and benefit of the interaction)
Behavior Change Counseling Index (BECCI; Lane et al. 2005)	11-item checklist with items rated on a 5-point Likert scale	Ratings in four domains of MI: agenda setting and permission seeking, the why and how of change in behavior, the whole consultation, talk about targets
Yale Adherence Competence Scale (YACS; Carroll et al. 2000)	50-item scale to assess elements common to all psychotherapies, with 9 additional MI-specific items	Three general ratings (assessment, general support, goals for treatment) and three specific ratings (clinical management, 12-step facilitation, cognitive-behavioral management); assessment of both adherence (how often a technique was used) and competence (how well the technique was executed)

TABLE 12–3. Tools to assess adherence and competence while implementing motivational interviewing (MI) intervention *(continued)*

Scale	What it consists of	What it measures
Independent Tape Rater Scale (ITRS)[b]	Adapted from the YACS; 39-item scale using 7-point Likert responses	Three ratings: MI-consistent interventions, MI-inconsistent interventions, and general substance abuse counseling interventions
Sequential Code for Observing Process Exchanges (SCOPE)[c]	Adapted from the MISC and Commitment Language Coding System (Amrhein et al. 2003), a sequential coding system focusing on client–therapist interaction, therapy process, and client outcome	Therapist behavior codes (including advise, affirm, confront, questions, reflect, etc.); client behavior codes (ask, commitment language, ability, need, reasons, taking steps)
Motivational Interviewing Supervision and Training Scale (MISTS; Madson et al. 2005)	Behavioral count of therapist responses and 16-item global ratings of quality, MI fidelity, and effectiveness of therapist interventions on 7-point Likert scale	Behavioral counts of therapist responses, including open questions and reflections, and 16 global ratings on aspects of MI (e.g., simple and complex reflection, rolling with resistance, MI spirit)
Motivational Interviewing Target Scheme (MITS 2.1; Allison et al. 2012)	Behavioral count of 10 therapist behaviors on a 4-point Likert scale	Behavioral counts of 10 therapist responses (e.g., activity emphasis, posture, empathy, collaboration)

TABLE 12–3. Tools to assess adherence and competence while implementing motivational interviewing (MI) intervention (*continued*)

Scale	What it consists of	What it measures
Video Assessment of Simulated Encounters—Revised (VASE-R; Rosengren et al. 2008)	18 items that produces a total score and five subscale scores of respondent skill in response to vignettes of simulated clients	Scoring of respondents' behaviors (reflective listening, responding to resistance, summarizing, eliciting change talk, and developing discrepancy)

[a]T.B. Moyers, J.K. Manuel, D. Ernst, "Motivational Interviewing Treatment Integrity Coding Manual 4.2.1," unpublished manual, June 2015).
[b]S.A. Ball, S. Martino, J. Corvino, et al., "Independent Tape Rater Guide," unpublished psychotherapy tape rating manual, New Haven, CT, Department of Psychiatry, Division of Substance Abuse, Yale School of Medicine, January 2002.
[c]T. Martin, T. B. Moyers, J. M. Houck, et al., "Motivational Interviewing Sequential Code for Observing Process Exchanges (MI-SCOPE) Coder's Manual," unpublished manuscript, Albuquerque, University of New Mexico, Center on Alcoholism, Substance Abuse, and Addictions, 2005. Available at: http://casaa.unm.edu/download/scope.pdf.

et al. 2007; Strang and McCambridge 2004). In assessing patient language, it may be necessary to audiotape or videotape sessions and use a formal coding system to assess the presence of change talk and sustain talk and/or the valence (positive or negative) of clinician reflections.

How Is Motivational Interviewing Different When Used Clinically and in Research?

This chapter has covered many aspects important in the science of MI. Research requires the ability to distinguish between MI and other types of interventions. In addition, there are many studies that have shown that MI is an effective intervention for a wide variety of problematic behaviors and symptoms. Regarding the use of MI in clinical practice versus research, one of the main differences is that research requires the delivery of a standardized intervention. Standardization means that all study clinicians are conducting the same intervention. This begins with comprehensive clinician training (both initial and ongoing) and evaluation to determine their competency. Some clinicians may not become proficient enough in MI to participate in the study, and MI can be time-consuming to learn. However, many people from various backgrounds have been successfully trained in MI. In addition to training, treatment fidelity must be ensured. In research, this is often measured by raters who complete standardized assessments but rarely provide feedback to study clinicians. Study clinicians usually receive intensive audiotaped or videotaped supervision throughout the study alongside ongoing, rigorous assessment of their performance.

In addition to differences in the delivery of the intervention, researchers usually examine change in groups of patients, as opposed to change in individual patients. In order to attribute change to the MI intervention, researchers often compare the MI intervention group with another group of patients who receive a different type of intervention (i.e., comparison group) or no intervention at all (i.e., control group). Research also requires special permission and oversight from institutional committees called Institutional Review Boards. These boards review all study procedures to make sure that patients who participate in the study will be treated ethically. Ethical treatment of research participants includes having each participant give informed consent and making sure that the potential benefits of participating in the study outweigh the risks. *Informed consent* means that participants know about study procedures, duration, and risks and benefits of being in the study. Finally, research differs from usual practice in the ability to share findings with a broader audience of clinicians and researchers.

CAN MOTIVATIONAL INTERVIEWING BE FAITHFULLY IMPLEMENTED IN REAL-WORLD SETTINGS?

Implementation science studies how promising research findings, developed under controlled conditions, translate into clinical practice and health care policy. This relatively new field of inquiry seeks to understand how the behavior of clinicians, administrators, and other stakeholders impacts the implementation of evidence-based interventions such as MI. The intention of implementation science is to identify and address the barriers (philosophical, social, behavioral, financial, and systems) that impede successful implementation in different settings and to test the effectiveness of novel therapeutic approaches in the real world where conditions are less controlled.

MI's efficacy for addiction and other problematic behaviors has been confirmed through a number of research studies (Lundahl and Burke 2009; Lundahl et al. 2010, 2013; Madson et al. 2016). As a result, clinicians, treatment facilities, and clinical training programs have become increasingly interested in this approach. That said, implementation of MI in nonresearch settings varies greatly, depending on the expertise of the interventionists and the level of institutional support provided. As mentioned in the section "How Do I Learn Motivational Interviewing?" in order for clinicians to learn MI, programs need to put forth a significant investment in initial training, as well as provide continued support and supervision from experts. This may be cost prohibitive for many treatment sites whose budgets are already quite limited and who may experience high levels of staff turnover. Because of concerns about the feasibility of training clinicians to deliver MI in real-world settings, some researchers are advocating for the development of new, briefer, accelerated training and supervision (Madson et al. 2016).

One alternative approach may be to train peers to provide MI interventions. There is some evidence that HIV-positive peers can be trained to deliver MI interventions, but the training required for peers to reach proficiency was more intensive compared with clinicians, and peers had difficulty adopting an MI communication style (e.g., reflective listening instead of giving advice) (Wolfe et al. 2013). Another potential alternative may be to incorporate technology in treatment delivery. A recent review of technology-delivered (e.g., Web-based, computer-delivered methodology) MI interventions reported that patients rated the acceptability and/or liking of these interventions very highly. In addition, the technology-delivered MI interventions were found to be generally efficacious; they worked to promote positive behavioral and psychological change (Shingleton and Palfai 2016). Given that technology-delivered interventions can provide cost-effective, easily accessible interventions with good fidelity (and limited clinician training, if applicable), technology-delivered MI interventions may be an attractive choice for programs that want to improve patient outcomes and minimize therapist costs and burden.

CONCLUSION

The science behind MI contains a number of important findings. MI is superior to no treatment and is equivalent to other active treatments despite its relative brevity. The measurement of intervention fidelity is growing among clinical trials, but it is still lacking in many trials that claim to use MI but do not present evidence of its competent use or fidelity to its spirit and methods. Last, the study of process-outcome relationships in MI is complex and ongoing. The how of MI is becoming clearer, with strong support for MI spirit being important in promoting positive change. There is more modest support for evoking change talk to promote positive change in patients, although the interplay among potential mechanisms and patient characteristics is complex. As more information about process-outcome relationships in MI accumulates, it will inform the development of an empirically based model of MI and, perhaps, of related psychotherapies.

REFERENCES

Acosta M, Haller DL, Ingersoll K: The science of motivational interviewing, in Handbook of Motivation and Change. Edited by Levounis P, Arnaout, B. Washington, DC, American Psychiatric Publishing, 2010, pp 237–254

Allison J, Bes R, Rose G: Motivational Interviewing Target Scheme (MITS 2.1): An Instrument for Practitioners, Trainers, Coaches and Researchers. Hilversum, The Netherlands, MiCampus, 2012

Alperstein D, Sharpe L: The efficacy of motivational interviewing in adults with chronic pain: a meta-analysis and systematic review. J Pain 17(4):393–403, 2016 26639413

Amrhein PC, Miller WR, Yahne CE, et al: Client commitment language during motivational interviewing predicts drug use outcomes. J Consult Clin Psychol 71(5):862–878, 2003 14516235

Apodaca TR, Longabaugh R: Mechanisms of change in motivational interviewing: a review and preliminary evaluation of the evidence. Addiction 104(5):705–715, 2009 19413785

Barnett E, Spruijt-Metz D, Moyers TB, et al: Bidirectional relationships between client and counselor speech: the importance of reframing. Psychol Addict Behav 28(4):1212–1219, 2014 24955660

Beck AT, Steer RA, Brown GK: Beck Depression Inventory. San Antonio, TX, Psychological Corporation, 1996

Blanchard KA, Morgenstern J, Morgan TJ, et al: Motivational subtypes and continuous measures of readiness for change: concurrent and predictive validity. Psychol Addict Behav 17(1):56–65, 2003 12665082

Brug J, Spikmans F, Aartsen C, et al: Training dietitians in basic motivational interviewing skills results in changes in their counseling style and in lower saturated fat intakes in their patients. J Nutr Educ Behav 39(1):8–12, 2007 17276321

Carroll KM, Nich C, Sifry RL, et al: A general system for evaluating therapist adherence and competence in psychotherapy research in the addictions. Drug Alcohol Depend 57(3):225–238, 2000 10661673

Cascaes AM, Bielemann RM, Clark VL, et al: Effectiveness of motivational interviewing at improving oral health: a systematic review. Rev Saude Publica 48(1):142–153, 2014 24789647

Clair-Michaud M, Martin RA, Stein LA, et al: The impact of motivational interviewing on delinquent behaviors in incarcerated adolescents. J Subst Abuse Treat 65:13–19, 2016 26517954

Copeland L, McNamara R, Kelson M, et al: Mechanisms of change within motivational interviewing in relation to health behaviors outcomes: a systematic review. Patient Educ Couns 98(4):401–411, 2015 25535015

Cushing CC, Jensen CD, Miller MB, et al: Meta-analysis of motivational interviewing for adolescent health behavior: efficacy beyond substance use. J Consult Clin Psychol 82(6):1212–1218, 2014 24841861

D'Amico EJ, Hunter SB, Miles JN, et al: A randomized controlled trial of a group motivational interviewing intervention for adolescents with a first time alcohol or drug offense. J Subst Abuse Treat 45(5):400–408, 2013 23891459

Dunn C, Deroo L, Rivara FP: The use of brief interventions adapted from motivational interviewing across behavioral domains: a systematic review. Addiction 96(12):1725–1742, 2001 11784466

Gao X, Lo EC, Kot SC, et al: Motivational interviewing in improving oral health: a systematic review of randomized controlled trials. J Periodontol 85(3):426–437, 2014 23805818

Gaston L, Marmar CR: The California Psychotherapy Alliance Scales, in The Working Alliance: Theory, Research, and Practice. Edited by Horvath AO, Greenberg LS. Oxford, UK, Wiley, 1994, pp 85–108

Glynn LH, Moyers TB: Chasing change talk: the clinician's role in evoking client language about change. J Subst Abuse Treat 39(1):65–70, 2010 20418049

Hatcher RL, Gillaspy JA: Development and validation of a revised short version of the Working Alliance Inventory. Psychother Res 16(1):12–25, 2006

Hettema J, Steele J, Miller WR: Motivational interviewing. Annu Rev Clin Psychol 1:91–111, 2005 17716083

Horvath AO, Greenberg L: Development and validation of the Working Alliance Inventory. J Couns Psychol 36(2):223–233, 1989

Hustad JT, Mastroleo NR, Kong L, et al: The comparative effectiveness of individual and group brief motivational interventions for mandated college students. Psychol Addict Behav 28(1):74–84, 2014 24731111

Jensen CD, Cushing CC, Aylward BS, et al: Effectiveness of motivational interviewing interventions for adolescent substance use behavior change: a meta-analytic review. J Consult Clin Psychol 79(4):433–440, 2011 21728400

Jones A, Gladstone BP, Lübeck M, et al: Motivational interventions in the management of HbA1c levels: a systematic review and meta-analysis. Prim Care Diabetes 8(2):91–100, 2014 24525286

Knight K, Holcom M, Simpson DD: TCU Psychosocial Functioning and Motivation Scales: Manual on Psychometric Properties. Fort Worth, Texas Christian University, Institute of Behavioral Research, 1994

Lane C, Huws-Thomas M, Hood K, et al: Measuring adaptations of motivational interviewing: the development and validation of the Behavior Change Counseling Index (BECCI). Patient Educ Couns 56(2):166–173, 2005 15653245

Larsen DL, Attkisson CC, Hargreaves WA, et al: Assessment of client/patient satisfaction: development of a general scale. Eval Program Plann 2(3):197–207, 1979 10245370

Luborsky L, Barber JP, Siqueland L, et al: The revised Helping Alliance Questionnaire (HAq-II): psychometric properties. J Psychother Pract Res 5(3):260–271, 1996 22700294

Lundahl B, Burke BL: The effectiveness and applicability of motivational interviewing: a practice-friendly review of four meta-analyses. J Clin Psychol 65(11):1232–1245, 2009 19739205

Lundahl BW, Kunz C, Brownell C, et al: A meta-analysis of motivational interviewing: twenty-five years of empirical studies. Res Soc Work Pract 20(2):137–160, 2010

Lundahl B, Moleni T, Burke BL, et al: Motivational interviewing in medical care settings: a systematic review and meta-analysis of randomized controlled trials. Patient Educ Couns 93(2):157–168, 2013 24001658

Macdonald P, Hibbs R, Corfield F, et al: The use of motivational interviewing in eating disorders: a systematic review. Psychiatry Res 200(1):1–11, 2012 22717144

Madson MB, Campbell TC, Barrett DE, et al: Development of the Motivational Interviewing Supervision and Training Scale. Psychol Addict Behav 19(3):303–310, 2005 16187810

Madson MB, Loignon AC, Lane C: Training in motivational interviewing: a systematic review. J Subst Abuse Treat 36(1):101–109, 2009 18657936

Madson MB, Schumacher JA, Baer JS, et al: Motivational interviewing for substance use: mapping out the next generation of research. J Subst Abuse Treat 65:1–5, 2016 26971078

Marsden J, Stillwell G, Barlow H, et al: An evaluation of a brief motivational intervention among young ecstasy and cocaine users: no effect on substance and alcohol use outcomes. Addiction 101(7):1014–1026, 2006 16771893

McConnaughy EA, Prochaska JO, Velicer WF: Stages of change in psychotherapy: measurement and sample profiles. Psychotherapy: Theory Research & Practice 20(3):368–375, 1982

McMurran M: Motivational interviewing with offenders: a systematic review. Legal and Criminological Psychology 14(1):83–100, 2009

Miller WR, Mount KA: A small study of training in motivational interviewing: does one workshop change clinician and patient behavior? Behav Cogn Psychother 29(4):457–471, 2001

Miller WR, Moyers TB: Eight stages in learning motivational interviewing. Journal of Teaching in the Addictions 5(1):3–17, 2006

Miller WR, Rollnick S: Motivational Interviewing: Preparing People for Change. New York, Guilford, 1991

Miller WR, Rollnick S: Motivational Interviewing: Helping People Change, 3rd Edition. New York, Guilford, 2013

Miller WR, Rose GS: Toward a theory of motivational interviewing. Am Psychol 64(6):527–537, 2009 19739882

Miller WR, Rose GS: Motivational interviewing and decisional balance: contrasting responses to client ambivalence. Behav Cogn Psychother 43(2):129–141, 2015 24229732

Miller WR, Tonigan JS: Assessing drinkers' motivation for change: the Stages of Change Readiness and Treatment Eagerness Scale (SOCRATES). Psychol Addict Behav 10(2):81–89, 1996

Miller WR, Yahne CE, Moyers TB, et al: A randomized trial of methods to help clinicians learn motivational interviewing. J Consult Clin Psychol 72(6):1050–1062, 2004 15612851

Morgenstern J, Kuerbis A, Amrhein P, et al: Motivational interviewing: a pilot test of active ingredients and mechanisms of change. Psychol Addict Behav 26(4):859–869, 2012 22905896

Moyers T, Martin T, Catley D, et al: Assessing the integrity of motivational interviewing interventions: reliability of the Motivational Interviewing Skills Code. Behav Cogn Psychother 31:177–184, 2003

Moyers TB, Martin T, Christopher PJ, et al: Client language as a mediator of motivational interviewing efficacy: where is the evidence? Alcohol Clin Exp Res 31(10 suppl):40s–47s, 2007 17880345

Moyers TB, Manuel JK, Ernst D: Motivational Interviewing Treatment Integrity Coding Manual 4.2.1, unpublished manual, June 2015

Prochaska JO, DiClemente CC: Stages and processes of self-change of smoking: toward an integrative model of change. J Consult Clin Psychol 51(3):390–395, 1983 6863699

Rosengren DB, Hartzler B, Baer JS, et al: The Video Assessment of Simulated Encounters—Revised (VASE-R): reliability and validity of a revised measure of motivational interviewing skills. Drug Alcohol Depend 97(1–2):130–138, 2008 18499356

Rubak S, Sandbaek A, Lauritzen T, et al: Motivational interviewing: a systematic review and meta-analysis. Br J Gen Pract 55(513):305–312, 2005 15826439

Saitz R, Palfai TP, Cheng DM, et al: Screening and brief intervention for drug use in primary care: the ASPIRE randomized clinical trial. JAMA 312(5):502–513, 2014 25096690

Schumacher JA, Madson MB, Nilsen P: Barriers to learning motivational interviewing: a survey of motivational interviewing trainers' perceptions. J Addict Offender Couns 35(2):81–96, 2014

Schwalbe CS, Oh HY, Zweben A: Sustaining motivational interviewing: a meta-analysis of training studies. Addiction 109(8):1287–1294, 2014 24661345

Shingleton RM, Palfai TP: Technology-delivered adaptations of motivational interviewing for health-related behaviors: a systematic review of the current research. Patient Educ Couns 99(1):17–35, 2016 26298219

Söderlund LL, Madson MB, Rubak S, et al: A systematic review of motivational interviewing training for general health care practitioners. Patient Educ Couns 84(1):16–26, 2011 20667432

Spencer JC, Wheeler SB: A systematic review of motivational interviewing interventions in cancer patients and survivors. Patient Educ Couns 99(7):1099–1105, 2016

Spohr SA, Taxman FS, Rodriguez M, et al: Motivational interviewing fidelity in a community corrections setting: treatment initiation and subsequent drug use. J Subst Abuse Treat 65:20–25, 2016 26365536

Strang J, McCambridge J: Can the practitioner correctly predict outcome in motivational interviewing? J Subst Abuse Treat 27(1):83–88, 2004 15223098

Substance Abuse and Mental Health Services Administration: Systems-level implementation of screening, brief intervention, and referral to treatment. Technical Assistance Publication Series 33. HHS Publication No (SMA) 13-4741. Rockville, MD, Substance Abuse and Mental Health Services Administration, 2013

Vasilaki EI, Hosier SG, Cox WM: The efficacy of motivational interviewing as a brief intervention for excessive drinking: a meta-analytic review. Alcohol Alcohol 41(3):328–335, 2006 16547122

Velicer WF, DiClemente CC, Prochaska JO, et al: Decisional balance measure for assessing and predicting smoking status. J Pers Soc Psychol 48(5):1279–1289, 1985 3998990

Velicer WF, Fava JL, Prochaska JO, et al: Distribution of smokers by stage in three representative samples. Prev Med 24(4):401–411, 1995 7479632

Wolfe H, Haller DL, Benoit E, et al: Developing PeerLink to engage out-of-care HIV+ substance users: training peers to deliver a peer-led motivational intervention with fidelity. AIDS Care 25(7):888–894, 2013 23230862

STUDENT REFLECTIONS

Mike Wang
Yale School of Medicine, MS3

As future clinicians, we need to recognize that implementation of evidence-based and standardized treatment in patient care is important for objective measurements of clinical change and thus provides a solid basis for feedback on how to improve one's own clinical performance. Evidence-based interventions also streamline economic analyses of medicine, and such streamlining is sorely needed in this era of soaring health care costs.

There is a broad base of evidence supporting the use of motivational interviewing (MI) as an effective treatment modality for a great variety of psychosocial problems in many different populations, such as reducing substance use in adolescents, improving health behaviors, managing lifestyle issues among cancer patients, and so forth. A caveat to this is that, although statistically significant, the effect size of MI is generally limited and the greatest efficacy is shown when MI is being compared to standard care or wait-list control groups, as opposed to other effective interventions. A potential reason for the modest effect size is the lack of standardization and rigor in MI implementation across studies, which needs to be further teased out in future studies.

Given the support in literature for MI as a relatively powerful tool for engendering positive behavioral change despite its relative brevity of delivery, it's almost certain that I, as a learner and future practitioner of medicine, will make use of MI for my patients. However, I think it's of paramount importance to undergo proper training in order to practice MI with fidelity, and continual supervision and feedback is needed in order to prevent drifting away from the evidence-based MI intervention. Further research and development is also needed to overcome the potentially prohibitive cost barrier of implementing rigorous and standardized MI in a real-world setting. The prospect of novel deliveries in MI interventions, such as peer-based or technology-delivered approaches, is also very exciting for the future of this evidence-based therapy.

Appendix 1 |

Key Concepts in Motivation and Change

FUNDAMENTALS OF MOTIVATIONAL INTERVIEWING (CHAPTER 2)

- Change is natural and intrinsic and can be hastened by a supportive yet directive approach.

- Motivational interviewing (MI) is an approach for developing the patient's intrinsic motivation for behavior change by using a style of communication that blends patient-centered listening skills with methods directed at eliciting the patient's motivation and commitment for change.

- The clinician adopts a spirit of interacting with the patient, marked by partnership, acceptance, compassion, and evocation of the patient's resources and motivations for change.

- MI happens in four overlapping processes that build on one another: engaging, focusing, evoking, and planning.

- MI core skills include use of fundamental patient-centered listening skills known as OARS (open questions, affirmations, reflections, and summaries) and giving information and advice in an MI-consistent manner.

- The clinician's ability to recognize and elicit change talk in the context of the spirit of the approach is the main mechanism by which MI is presumed to work.

- MI has many parallels with other modes of therapy, and the ability to provide change-oriented therapy is seen as common to many schools of psychotherapy.

- Teaching and supervision are effectively done in a supportive and collaborative manner that is consistent with the spirit of MI. Skills can be mastered and applied with adequate instruction and supervision. Change in trainees is natural.

ENGAGING (CHAPTER 3)

Goals of Engaging

1. Ensure the patient participates in treatment.

2. Help the patient feel safe to share information.

3. Allow the patient to feel understood, respected, and trusted.

4. Allow the patient to participate in a collaborative way.

Behaviors That Support Engagement

1. Practicing good listening.

2. Providing undivided attention.

3. Comforting with eye contact and genuine facial expression.

Traps to Avoid

1. Excessive questioning.

2. Hierarchical dyad between patient and clinician.

3. Prematurely labeling a patient's problem.

4. Judging and blaming the patient.

5. Excessive chatting.

OARS: Fundamentals of Engaging

Open questions: "How has it been for you since we last met? [*Broad, inviting the patient to elaborate*].

Affirming: "It is great that you think about your family." [*Genuine, pointing out the positive, acknowledging strength and values.*]

Reflecting: Simple reflection: "Strong cravings" [*Repeating or rephrasing what the patient says*]; Complex reflections: "You are struggling with the cravings" [*Providing an educated guess about the meaning, context, or feeling associated with what the patient said*].

Summarizing: "You had increased stress, and it triggered your cravings, which led to you having a couple of drinks. It was good that you returned to the group, to get back on track. Your family is important to you, and you want to continue to work on your sobriety." [*Clear, concise overview, with affirmations and reflections, ending on a positive note.*]

FOCUSING (CHAPTER 4)

- There are three sources of focus: the patient, the setting, and the clinician. There are three common focusing scenarios:

  1. Focus and direction are clear.

  2. There are several choices to focus on (the focus is not clear).

  3. There is no clear focus (the direction is unclear).

- Start with orienting and once a few options come into view, you can use the following strategies to get the focus to become clearer:

  - Agenda mapping

  - Zooming in

  - Elicit-provide-elicit

  - Changing direction

- Keep in mind the four aspects of the spirit of MI when focusing: partnership, acceptance, compassion, and evocation.

EVOKING (CHAPTER 5)

- The mnemonic DARN CAT can be very helpful for remembering the various types of change talks:

  - Desire

  - Ability

  - Reasons

  - Need

  - Commitment

- Activation
- Taking steps
- The mnemonic OARS can be very helpful in remembering responsive skills that serve to reinforce and facilitate change talk:
  - Open questions
  - Affirmation
  - Reflection
  - Summaries
- Recognize
  - Ambivalence
  - Change talk (preparatory [DARN]/mobilizing [CAT])
  - Sustain talk (DARN CAT)
  - Discord (defensiveness, squaring off, interrupting, disengagement)
- Respond
  - Change talk (OARS)
  - Sustain talk (reflect and strategize)
  - Discord (reflect, strategize, apologize, affirm, redirect)
- Evoke
  - Change (questions, importance ruler, extremes, looking back/looking forward)
  - Confidence (talk, confidence ruler, review past successes, hypotheticals)
  - Motivation (discrepancy, exchanging information, others' concerns)
- Remembering acronyms and visualizing conceptual metaphors can aid in providing more salient memories of MI.
- The ruler is a conceptual metaphor that you can utilize to help evoke change talk. Imagine a ruler, which has been numbered 0 to 10. Next, ask the patient to rate the importance of change. Whatever number they report, ask them why a lower number was not chosen and reflect change talk. If the number is 0, then ask what it would take for the number to increase. The same technique can be used in evoking confidence.

PLANNING (CHAPTER 6)

When Should Planning Begin?

* *Signs of readiness:* increased ratio of change to sustain talk, strengthening change talk statements, planning for change.

* *Testing the water:* present a "bouquet" of change talk (recapitulation); ask the key question "What would you like to do next?"

Creating a Robust Change Plan

* The best plans are clear and precise.

* SMART Goals: Specific, measurable, action-oriented, realistic, and time-bound. Change planning should remain collaborative—maintain the motivational interviewing (MI) spirit.

If Commitment Diminishes

* Remember that fluctuating commitment is normal in the process of change.

* Listen for and support any residual mobilizing change talk.

* Ask, "What else might help you commit to your change goal?"

* Break the change plan down into smaller, more achievable steps.

* Consider useful suggestions (with permission) such as self-monitoring and enlisting the support of a significant other.

As the Plan Is Being Implemented

* Support the change being made (this is essential).

* Avoid pejorative language and dichotomous ("black and white") thinking about goals.

* Encourage: catch setbacks early and normalize the nonlinear nature of change.

* Consider revisiting the other MI processes in supporting change.

Remember that MI can be integrated with other therapeutic approaches.

INTEGRATING MOTIVATIONAL INTERVIEWING WITH OTHER PSYCHOTHERAPIES (CHAPTER 7)

- Motivational interviewing (MI) can be woven into other psychotherapy modalities using either a *sequenced* or a *combined* approach.

- *Sequenced* approaches consist of using two or more psychotherapy techniques in an alternating manner. These approaches are most useful when the clinician is addressing low motivation in the context of a psychotherapeutic modality other than MI. Examples include
  - Using an MI prelude prior to starting cognitive-behavioral therapy (CBT) to enhance motivation and to establish a strong therapeutic alliance.

  - Inserting a piece of MI to address homework noncompliance during CBT.

  - Using an MI-informed approach to address relapse to substance use during the course of psychodynamic therapy (or other modalities).

- *Combined* approaches to integration blend elements of MI within the framework of a second form of psychotherapy to form a synergistic whole. Examples include
  - Using OARS (open questions, affirmations, reflections, summaries) skills to enhance forward momentum in the context of supportive psychotherapy that targets behavioral change.

  - Using open-ended questions and reflective statements to explore ambivalence about pursuing treatment modalities and resources (e.g., pharmacotherapy, Alcoholics Anonymous attendance).

  - Using affirmations to enhance self-esteem, which is a core goal of supportive psychotherapy.

  - Asking for permission or using the elicit-provide-elicit approach to promote a sense of collaboration when giving advice in the context of supportive psychotherapy.

- MI can be delivered in a group format. Important tasks to consider when doing so include
  - Educating group members about the spirit of MI.

  - Intervening promptly when MI-inconsistent behaviors occur.

- Balancing group and individual interventions.
- Maximizing change talk.

MOTIVATIONAL INTERVIEWING AND PHARMACOTHERAPY (CHAPTER 8)

- Motivational interviewing (MI) is a useful approach when incorporating pharmacotherapy into treatment.
  1. Engaging.
     a. Resist the assessment trap.
     b. Use open questions to discover what the patient understands to be the issue.
     c. Do not assume.
  2. Focusing.
     a. Identify the patient's goals and how medications align with achieving them.
     b. Build on information and experience from the past; collaborate on a plan for the future.
     c. Elicit what the patient knows about treatment. After asking permission, provide data about evidence-based treatment and medications in a transparent and factual manner. Elicit understanding and incorporation of newly provided information.
  3. Evoking.
     a. Though medications are an important component of treatment and their utility is supported by evidence, there are many factors that limit their broad utilization.
     b. Appreciate that there are negatives to taking medications.
     c. Evoke change talk for taking medications.
     d. Support self-efficacy.
  4. Planning.
     a. Offer a menu of options.
     b. Collaborate with the patient to formulate a plan of action for taking medication.

   c. Address barriers to treatment, help increase commitment to change, and continue to strengthen therapeutic alliance to increase adherence.

5. Support patient actions.

   a. Utilize evidence-based pharmacotherapies and provide information in a nonjudgmental, clear manner.

6. Ask about adherence.

   a. Use MI to foster an open discussion about potential issues of adherence, which are often complex and multifactorial.

   b. Acknowledge that adherence is difficult and periodically ask whether the patient is experiencing any problems taking his or her medication.

   c. Affirm any reduction of an undesired behavior and reflect upon it in the context of the patient's goals.

   d. If a patient experiences a return to use, use it as an opportunity to explore the patient's ambivalence rather than view it as a failure of treatment.

MOTIVATIONAL INTERVIEWING IN A DIVERSE SOCIETY (CHAPTER 9)

- Motivational interviewing (MI) is used throughout the world in numerous languages.

- There is robust evidence to support the effectiveness of MI in adolescents, and some evidence to suggest that MI has some positive effect in geriatric populations.

- There is some evidence to suggest that racial/ethnic concordance of the MI clinician and patient/client enhances the efficacy of MI.

- MI that judiciously incorporates cultural norms can improve the engagement phase of the interview.

- There is no evidence that MI has more or less effect in lesbian, gay, bisexual, and transgender (LGBT) patients than in the general population.

- MI's emphasis on partnership, acceptance (including autonomy), compassion, and evocation supports clinicians working with LGBT patients, where openness can help avoid misplaced assumptions.

- Good clinicians should be reasonably free of homophobia, transphobia, and heterosexism; have positive regard for the patient; welcome and promote openness about sexual orientation and gender identity in the therapeutic setting; and be familiar with many of the issues commonly faced by LGBT persons.

- MI is congruent with structurally competent care.

TEACHING MOTIVATIONAL INTERVIEWING (CHAPTER 10)

- Teaching motivational interviewing (MI) is an excellent opportunity to use the spirit of MI and to model the four processes of MI as the framework for doing the training. Teaching strategies include didactic and experiential learning followed by supervision, monitoring, and feedback.

- In addition to the four processes of MI used to frame teaching, another useful framework is informed by the Gradual Release of Responsibility Model, commonly understood as the "I do it, we do it, you do it" model, that can be consistent with the MI style.

- Several activities have been developed to help trainees learn or practice the four MI processes or various MI skills and techniques that can be found in this chapter and in MI training materials available at www.motivationalinterviewing.org. There are also many video demonstrations of both MI-consistent and MI-inconsistent encounters that can illustrate many points and that are useful to vary teaching methodologies.

- Although the MI training session may end, it is helpful to think about learning MI as a perpetual process of training, skill practice, supervision, reflection, and refinement.

MOTIVATIONAL INTERVIEWING IN ADMINISTRATION, MANAGEMENT, AND LEADERSHIP (CHAPTER 11)

- Motivational interviewing (MI) concepts, developed to facilitate change in individuals, can be applied to changing the culture of systems composed of individuals.

- When using the transtheoretical model, apply the following:
  1. In the precontemplation stage, plant the seed of ambivalence.
  2. In the contemplation stage, explore both the positive and the negative prospects of life with and without the proposed change in culture.
  3. In the preparation stage, develop a realistic action plan that anticipates problems and identifies solutions.
  4. During the action stage, consolidate intrinsic motivation with extrinsic coercion.
  5. In the maintenance stage, use a multitude of motivational and psychosocial approaches to sustain the desired change.
  6. If relapse occurs, accept it as an opportunity to reengage, rethink, and reemerge stronger than before.
- When using the four-processes model, implement the following:
  1. Engage people on mutually negotiated and agreed-upon goals and potentially the tasks required to reach these goals.
  2. Focus on pursuing and upholding a direction of change, while tolerating the uncertainty intrinsic to change.
  3. Evoke change talk and manage sustain talk. Develop discrepancies, foster motivation, and resolve ambivalence.
  4. Plan for the long run by setting up achievable, yet gradually challenging, goals.
  5. Throughout the process, celebrate communication, collaboration, and the intrinsic motivation of individuals.

Appendix 2

Answer Guide to Study Questions

CHAPTER 2: FUNDAMENTALS OF MOTIVATIONAL INTERVIEWING

1. Motivational interviewing (MI) is most closely related to

   A. Psychoanalysis.
   B. Behaviorism.
   C. Humanistic psychology.
   D. The 12-step tradition.

   Correct Answer: C (Humanistic psychology).

   MI is deeply grounded in humanistic psychology, especially Carl Rogers's client-centered approach.

2. The spirit of MI lies in

   A. Criticism, elucidation, diagnosis, and analysis.
   B. Creativity, expansion, passivity, and advocacy.
   C. Confrontation, criticism, education, and authority.
   D. Partnership, acceptance, compassion, and evocation.

   Correct Answer: D (Partnership, acceptance, compassion, and evocation).

   In motivational interviewing clinicians honor the patient's experiences and perspective (partnership); affirm the patient's right and capacity for self-direction (acceptance); seek the patient's best interest (compassion), and draw out the patient's goals, values, and perceptions that support change (evocation).

3. Which of the following patient statements best predicts his or her readiness and commitment to change?

    A. "If I don't stop drinking, my liver cirrhosis will only get worse."
    B. "Last week I began leaving my cigarettes in the trunk of my car while driving so I wouldn't be tempted to smoke."
    C. "I could go for a walk after dinner instead of smoking a cigarette."
    D. "I desperately want to be able to fall asleep without needing a marijuana joint."

Correct Answer: B ("Last week I began leaving my cigarettes in the trunk of my car while driving so I wouldn't be tempted to smoke").

Although all of these statements represent change talk, only B is mobilizing change talk (taking steps), which indicates mobilization toward change. The other options are preparatory change talk indicating need (answer A), ability (answer C), and desire (answer D).

4. MI often can be successfully combined with other therapeutic modalities. This statement is

    A. False, because any association with other therapies will confuse the patient.
    B. True, because MI is compatible with many approaches.
    C. Dangerous, because therapists should always be passionate advocates of only one psychotherapeutic school.
    D. Irrelevant, because competent therapists spontaneously know what to do without the need to learn MI.

Correct Answer: B (True, because MI is compatible with many approaches).

MI is consistent with many other psychotherapeutic modalities and can be used as a prelude to them, a permeating factor used alongside other approaches, or a fallback position whenever motivational issues reemerge in treatment.

5. Teaching and supervision of MI

    A. Are best done in an accepting and collaborative manner.
    B. Are best done through confrontation to emphasize contrast with the style of MI.

C. Require that the student undergo his or her own motivational therapy.
D. Should focus on convincing the student that MI is better than other therapies.

Correct Answer: A (Are best done in an accepting and collaborative manner).

Teaching and supervision are best done in a supportive and collaborative manner that is consistent with the spirit of MI.

CHAPTER 3: ENGAGING

1. Engaging can be considered as

A. One of the stages of change.
B. An optional part of motivational interviewing (MI), only necessary for the most difficult patients.
C. An essential characteristic of the clinician, but does not involve the patient.
D. One of the four processes in MI, the foundation of every therapeutic relationship.
E. The end of therapy and is not a prerequisite for the other processes in MI.

Correct Answer: D (One of the four processes in MI, the foundation of every therapeutic relationship).

Engaging is not related to the stages of change. Engaging is an integral part of MI with all patients, not only difficult or vulnerable patients. The engagement process is started at the beginning of MI and should be reinforced throughout the partnership.

2. Which statement is *true* about the core communication skills in MI?

A. Closed questions should be applied more than open questions.
B. Open questions promote exploration and facilitate the natural flow of conversation.
C. A reflection is a core communication skill, but should be used minimally.
D. Summarizing refers to a compilation of all the flaws and deficits a patient may have.
E. Affirming is a strategy for depressed patients, to make them feel better.

Correct Answer: B (Open questions promote exploration and facilitate the natural flow of conversation).

A clinician should aim to favor more open questions than closed questions. Reflections are a helpful communication aid that should be used as often as needed. Summarizing involves reflections and affirmations and should not contain patient flaws. Affirmations should be genuine and aim to accentuate positive findings from the patient's behavioral repertoire. The goal is to make the patient feel valued and respected.

3. Of the following statements or questions, which one would best promote engagement?

    A. "Your urine toxicology was positive; where did you get the cocaine?"
    B. "I do not think you care about your sobriety. Look at your urine—it's positive."
    C. "I noticed some changes in your urine toxicology this week. Please tell me more about that."
    D. "Your daughter will be disappointed."
    E. "You broke your promise again."

Correct Answer: C ("I noticed some changes in your urine toxicology this week. Please tell me more about that").

When facing a positive unexpected urine toxicology finding, any judgmental language should be avoided. Simply stating the finding and providing an open question to explore more is consistent with the MI spirit and promotes engagement. A curious, genuinely concerned clinician is more likely to engage with a patient.

4. Which statement about affirmations is *true*?

    A. They do not have to be genuine.
    B. They are useful only when the patient is considering terminating the treatment.
    C. Many should be used in the interview, to make sure the patient likes the clinician.
    D. They should be used only after judging the patient for their behaviors.
    E. They are genuine and can acknowledge the strengths, values, and inherent worth of patients.

Correct Answer: E (They are genuine and can acknowledge the strengths, values, and inherent worth of patients).

Good affirmations are genuine, are useful throughout the engagement process, and do not have judgmental language. The goal is to validate the patient's strengths and values.

5. Which statement below best describes summarizing?

   A. It should not include reflections.
   B. It should not include affirmations.
   C. It has to be done only when terminating with a patient.
   D. It should be provided in a written format.
   E. It includes reflections and affirmations and allows the patient to clarify.

Correct Answer: E (It includes reflections and affirmations and allows the patient to clarify).

Summarizing throughout the engaging process includes the use of reflections and affirmations and allows the patient to clarify, if necessary. Summarizing is a core skill of MI and promotes engagement. It should not be reserved for later stages in therapy.

CHAPTER 4: FOCUSING

1. Which strategy is used when the patient has a goal that is far from the goal the clinician would like to discuss?

   A. Elicit-provide-elicit.
   B. Changing direction.
   C. Agenda mapping.
   D. Zooming in.
   E. Orienting.

Correct Answer: B (Changing direction).

Changing direction is used when there is a difference in goals between the patient and clinician.

2. A 30-year-old women presents to your office stating her life is completely in shambles. Which of the following is a technique to use in focusing during motivational interviewing (MI)?

   A. Zooming in.
   B. Imagining.

    C. Helping.
    D. Zoning out.
    E. Picturing.

Correct Answer: A (Zooming in).

Zooming in and zooming out are used when the patient has no specific goal. The clinician orients the patient first and can then zoom in to focus on a topic and navigate. When the need arises to orient again, the clinician can help by zooming out to review the bigger picture.

3. Which of the following questions can begin the process of agenda mapping?

    A. What is your psychiatric history?
    B. What is the chronological timeline for your presenting problem?
    C. Can you draw a few circles and write what you would like to discuss today?
    D. Where did we end the session last week?
    E. What would you like to talk about today?

Correct Answer: C (Can you draw a few circles and write what you would like to discuss today?).

Agenda mapping can be done as a visual aid to help the patient organize which topics they would like to focus on.

4. Which of the following scenarios would be considered unethical use of motivational interviewing (MI)?

    A. The patient has no focus and tells you a story that is very difficult to follow.
    B. The patient does not want to change.
    C. You are offered money in exchange for your clinical expertise.
    D. A CEO asks you to use MI to help bring patients to an intensive outpatient program in exchange for a medical directorship.
    E. A doctor consults you to talk to a diabetic patient about his poorly controlled blood glucose.

Correct Answer: D (A CEO asks you to use MI to help bring patients to an intensive outpatient program in exchange for a medical directorship).

This scenario represents a conflict of interest.

5. How does agenda mapping help the clinician using MI?

   A. Makes your life easier.
   B. Allows you to pick something quickly.
   C. Helps the clinician map out the session.
   D. Helps the clinician understand the breadth of possible agendas on which the patient may want to focus the conversation.
   E. Gives insight into the psyche of the patient.

Correct Answer: D (Helps the clinician understand the breadth of possible agendas upon which the patient may want to focus the conversation).

Agenda mapping is a strategy that can help the patient and clinician map out possible agendas on which they can focus in the interview.

CHAPTER 5: EVOKING

1. Which evoking question is most likely to inspire change talk?

   A. Why are you drinking daily?
   B. Why not stop drinking?
   C. What are you thinking?
   D. What's the downside of drinking alcohol?

Correct Answer: D (What's the downside of drinking alcohol?).

Exploring reasons for change can inspire preparatory change talk.

2. If you hear someone engaging in sustain talk, which of the following choices is the best response?

   A. Reframe.
   B. Affirm.
   C. Square off.
   D. Disengage.

Correct Answer: A (Reframe).

Reframing sustain talk is an excellent way to facilitate change in one's perception, which may lead to behavioral change.

3. Which of the following choices may worsen interpersonal discord?

   A. Apologize.
   B. Affirm.
   C. Square off.
   D. Redirect.

   Correct Answer: C (Square off).

   Squaring off will most likely further the discord and worsen the therapeutic alliance.

4. Which type of response is most likely to lead to sustain talk?

   A. Reflecting statement.
   B. Closed question.
   C. Affirmation.
   D. Summarizing statement.

   Correct Answer: B (Closed question).

   Whereas open questions lend themselves to more expansive answers and change talk, closed questions will likely lead to sustain talk.

5. Which of the following choices is an example of mobilizing change talk?

   A. Desire to change.
   B. Reasons to change.
   C. Ability to change.
   D. Commitment to change.

   Correct Answer: D (Commitment to change).

   Commitment to change is an example of mobilizing change talk. The other choices are examples of preparatory change talk.

CHAPTER 6: PLANNING

1. You've been working with a patient to cut down on drinking for the past 2 months. Recently, he has been late to appointments and has canceled a few times. When you do meet, he reveals that his drinking has been increasing. What stage of motivational interviewing (MI) is the most appropriate to revisit at this time?

  A. Replanning.
  B. Reevoking ("reminding").
  C. Refocusing.
  D. Reengaging.
  E. None; this patient's care should be transferred to another clinician.

Correct Answer: D (Reengaging).

Late and canceled appointments, as well as increasing substance abuse, are signs that the patient is disengaging. Remember, patients often do not reach their goal by way of a linear path straight through the processes of MI. Flagging engagement can be a natural part of the work, particularly when a sustained effort is required. While it may be necessary to eventually revisit several of the processes with this patient, at this point reengaging is most likely to help him start investing the necessary time and effort to achieve change.

2. *Recapitulation* refers to

  A. Repeating the patient's change talk back to them verbatim.
  B. Mirroring the patient's body language.
  C. Making a summary statement of collected change talk.
  D. One of the four fundamental processes of MI.
  E. The process of creating a change plan.

Correct Answer: C (Making a summary statement of collected change talk).

Recapitulation is an essential component of testing the water, a technique to gauge when a patient is ready to begin planning. Recapitulation consists of gathering up all the most powerful change talk statements from previous sessions and presenting them to the patient in a summary statement, or a "bouquet" of change talk. To complete the testing-the-water technique, the recapitulation is followed by a key question such as "How might you want to proceed from here?"

3. The "SMART" in SMART goals can stand for

  A. Sensible, maintainable, attune, resistance, two-part.
  B. Specific, measurable, action-oriented, realistic, time-bound.
  C. Serviceable, multiple, attached, richly developed, traditional.
  D. Stages, most-rewarding, autonomous, referenced, tolerable.
  E. Support, mindful, accurate, responsible, theoretical.

Correct Answer: B (Specific, measurable, action-oriented, realistic, time-bound).

Although multiple versions of the SMART goal mnemonic exist, specific, measurable, action-oriented, realistic, and time-bound is the only one of the choices presented that embodies the concept of SMART goals. Goals that are consistent with SMART are specific and quantifiable goals that can be realistically achieved through action.

4. Your patient is in the process of implementing a well-designed change plan but is having trouble achieving the goals she has set for herself. What might be the most useful next step?

   A. Advise her on strategies that you think might be helpful.
   B. Tell her that she needs to make a more sustained effort.
   C. Break down the change plan into smaller, more achievable intermediate goals.
   D. Be realistic and realize that she probably will not be able to achieve lasting change; helping her come to terms with this now will minimize disappointment in the end.
   E. Introduce her to another patient who achieved a similar goal.

Correct Answer: C (Break down the change plan into smaller, more achievable intermediate goals).

An inability to achieve previously set goals may be due to the fact that the goal is simply too ambitious to be done all at once. A good strategy is to examine the goal with the patient and work together to formulate smaller discrete steps toward the ultimate goal.

5. Which of the following statements represents mobilizing change talk for a patient trying to quit smoking?

   A. "I bought a box of nicotine patches yesterday and put one on for the first time this morning."
   B. "The cravings for cigarettes can be so powerful sometimes."
   C. "I know that smoking is bad for my health."
   D. "My family is always giving me a hard time about smoking. I really hope that I'm able to kick this habit!"
   E. "I could buy a car with the amount of money I spend on cigarettes."

Correct Answer: A ("I bought a box of nicotine patches yesterday and put one on for the first time this morning").

Mobilizing change talk is summarized by the CAT portion of the DARN CAT mnemonic. CAT stands for commitment, activation, and taking steps. A patient trying to quit smoking who buys nicotine patches is someone who has begun taking steps toward change.

CHAPTER 7: INTEGRATING MOTIVATIONAL INTERVIEWING WITH OTHER PSYCHOTHERAPIES

1. Which of the following psychotherapy integration approaches was Carl Rogers a proponent of?

   A. Theoretical integration.
   B. Common factors.
   C. Assimilative integration.
   D. Additive combining.
   E. Technical eclecticism.

   Correct Answer: B (Common factors).

   Carl Rogers's person-centered psychology resonates with the common factors approach in that he believed that certain therapist-specific factors are responsible for catalyzing patients' personal growth. These common factors consist of accurate empathy, unconditional positive regard, and self-congruence.

2. The first session of cognitive-behavioral therapy (CBT) for substance use disorders overlaps most with which motivational interviewing (MI) process?

   A. Engaging.
   B. Focusing.
   C. Evoking.
   D. Planning.
   E. Concluding.

   Correct Answer: D (Planning).

   The first session of CBT for substance use disorders makes use of core MI principles to enhance motivation for change while beginning to plan how the patient's goals can be achieved. This is analogous to the planning stage of MI, in which the therapist continues to strengthen commitment to change by using OARS (open questions, affirmations, reflections, summaries) skills while working with the patient toward developing a change plan. The other MI processes occur *before* the active planning stage. Option E is not an MI process.

3. The spirit of MI is most consistent with which of the following?

     A. Freudian drive theory.
     B. Object relations theory.
     C. Humanistic psychology.
     D. Self psychology.
     E. Attachment theory.

Correct Answer: C (Humanistic psychology).

The spirit of MI has roots in humanistic psychology, which posits that humans will move in the direction of positive change if the right conditions are present. These conditions are achieved when a therapist practices according to the spirit of MI. The spirit of MI comprises four elements: partnership, acceptance, compassion, and evocation.

4. Which of the following MI techniques is most helpful for giving advice to patients during a course of supportive psychotherapy?

     A. Reframe-remind-return.
     B. Complex reflective statements.
     C. Amplified reflections.
     D. Inform-reframe-inform.
     E. Elicit-provide-elicit.

Correct Answer: E (Elicit-provide-elicit).

The elicit-provide-elicit approach allows the therapist to share important information with the patient without coming across as authoritative, thus supporting patient autonomy. Answers B and C are techniques that may also be used in the course of supportive psychotherapy, but they are not specific to advice giving. Answer A refers to a technique used in group therapy to steer the group discussion back on track when MI-inconsistent behaviors occur.

5. Which of the following statements is *true* regarding MI delivered in a group setting?

     A. The therapist should use reflections to amplify "solution talk" by group members.
     B. MI delivered in groups is as efficacious as individually delivered MI.
     C. Group members should all be in the same "stage of change."
     D. Therapists should strive to maximize mobilizing change talk for each group member.
     E. Each group session should focus on one to two group members.

Correct Answer: D (Therapists should strive to maximize mobilizing change talk for each group member).

Change talk should be maximized in both group and individually delivered MI, because it has been directly correlated with behavior change. The other options are incorrect, given that "solution talk" is considered to be inconsistent with the spirit of MI, group MI has not been shown to be as effective as individual MI, and having a heterogeneous group with respect to stages of change is to be expected and can enhance group process by allowing members to learn from one another.

CHAPTER 8: MOTIVATIONAL INTERVIEWING AND PHARMACOTHERAPY

1. Why is motivational interviewing (MI) helpful in facilitating the use of medications?

   A. MI allows the patient to decide what they want to do, without the provider's input.
   B. It affords the opportunity to collaboratively build on information and experience from the past, leading to higher rates of success.
   C. It is not helpful in facilitating the use of medications in therapy.
   D. It allows the provider to list all of the reasons why the patient should take the medication, without interference with the patient's theoretical concerns.
   E. It allows the patient to be heard but ultimately relies on the provider's expertise to decide what is best.

   Correct Answer: B (It affords the opportunity to collaboratively build on information and experience from the past, leading to higher rates of success).

   This is the only option that incorporates the input of both the provider and the patient while defaulting to the patient's right to choose his or her treatment.

2. After completing alcohol detoxification, a patient is interested in a medication to help him quit. He has never attempted to stop drinking before, but the need for hospitalization has really scared him. His laboratory results are significant for abnormally elevated liver function tests. Renal function is normal. What would you recommend?

   A. Disulfiram.
   B. Naltrexone.

C. Acamprosate.

D. Extended-release naltrexone.

E. Alprazolam.

Correct Answer: C (Acamprosate).

The best option is likely to recheck and start naltrexone when liver function test results are lower. However, if the patient prefers the use of medication at this visit, consider acamprosate.

3. A patient says he wants to take medications to get better, but you call the pharmacy and discover he hasn't picked up his medications in months. What do you do?

   A. Nothing—see if he says anything at the next appointment.
   B. Discuss your discovery with the patient in a nonjudgmental and supportive way.
   C. Call the patient immediately and demand answers.
   D. Ask the patient to come in, ask open-ended questions, and, if he is amenable, restart medications with additional supports.
   E. Options B and D.

Correct Answer: E (Options B and D).

Use MI to talk with patients about their nonadherence and determine next steps, and make sure to check in on their confidence in following through.

4. A patient has experienced a return to use of alcohol despite taking naltrexone and attending weekly therapy. What do you do?

   A. Express your disappointment and ask the patient how she would like to proceed.
   B. Call the patient's family.
   C. Decide to no longer treat the patient, who probably wasn't really being compliant with the therapy, and refer her elsewhere.
   D. Use the return as an opportunity to discuss triggers for relapse, and collaborate on next steps.
   E. Tell the patient that this isn't working and that she has to go to a higher level of care.

Correct Answer: D (Use the return as an opportunity to discuss triggers for relapse, and collaborate on next steps).

It's imperative to be nonjudgmental and reinforce your commitment to the patient during a return to use. Although the patient may need a higher level of care or family support, this should be discussed first before any action is taken.

5. A patient says that she has been using 120 mg of oxycodone daily for the past 2 years. She was initially prescribed oxycodone for a back injury but quickly began using more than prescribed. She says she would like to be detoxed. What is the next step?

   A. Detox the patient.
   B. Say you do not recommend detox and tell her you will only treat her with buprenorphine.
   C. Refer the patient to a methadone clinic.
   D. Ask, "What do you know about maintenance treatment for opioid addiction?"
   E. Ask the patient how committed she is to treatment.

   Correct Answer: D (Ask, "What do you know about maintenance treatment for opioid addiction?").

   The recommended treatment for opioid use disorder is maintenance treatment with either buprenorphine/naloxone or methadone. Detoxification is not recommended, given the high rates of relapse and increased risk of overdose. In an MI-consistent manner, share this recommendation with the patient by first eliciting what she knows.

CHAPTER 9: MOTIVATIONAL INTERVIEWING IN A DIVERSE SOCIETY

1. How would you best describe the evidence that motivational interviewing (MI) supports adolescents changing their drug- or alcohol-related behaviors?

   A. The evidence is mixed (some studies show an effect, and other studies show no effect.
   B. The evidence is consistently positive (a strong positive effect).
   C. The evidence shows overwhelming harm (a strong detrimental effect).
   D. The evidence consistently shows no effect on drug or alcohol use in adolescents.

   Correct Answer: A (The evidence is mixed [some studies show an effect, and other studies show no effect]).

The evidence does not support that MI is always positive, is harmful, or lacks any effect on adolescents.

2. How does the effect of MI with racial and ethnic minorities in the United States compare with the effect shown in the general population?

    A. MI has been shown to be more harmful to racial and ethnic minorities.
    B. MI has been shown to have a stronger positive effect with racial and ethnic minorities.
    C. MI consistently works no better or worse.
    D. MI always requires the patient/client and clinician to be of the same race/ethnicity to show any benefit.

Correct Answer: B (MI has been shown to have a stronger positive effect with racial and ethnic minorities).

A 2005 U.S.-based meta-analysis found that MI effects were larger for ethnic minority populations, especially Native American groups. The other answers are not true. While MI among racially concordant clinicians and patients/clients may show a stronger effect as compared with discordant interviews, this difference is not always found, and MI has been shown to have benefits between clinicians and patients/clients of different races. MI has not been shown to be harmful in comparison with other therapies, and it has not consistently been shown to have an equivalent effect between racially concordant and discordant clinicians and patients/clients.

3. In which of the following situations was MI shown to have the strongest effect?

    A. When Native Americans are asked directly about their spiritual practices.
    B. When African American patients/clients are working with African American clinicians.
    C. When the clinician and patient/client share subtle cultural familiarities and nonverbal cues.
    D. When MI is provided in strict accordance with a manual.

Correct Answer: C (When the clinician and patient/client share subtle cultural familiarities and nonverbal cues).

Among Native American and Hispanic populations, MI has been postulated to work better when the clinician and patient/client share subtle cultural familiarities and nonverbal cues. Racial concordance among African

Americans between provider and patient/client has not been shown to increase MI's effectiveness. Asking Native Americans directly about spiritual practices and strictly following a manual are associated with poorer outcomes.

4. What has the majority of MI research involving gay and bisexual men focused on?

   A. Cigarette smoking.
   B. Eating behaviors.
   C. Alcohol use.
   D. HIV risk behaviors.

Correct Answer: D (HIV risk behaviors).

Among the studies of MI in populations of men who have sex with men, most have focused on HIV risk behaviors. Alcohol has been a secondary focus, and there are no studies of MI to date focused on tobacco use or eating behaviors in men who have sex with men.

5. Determining which gender pronouns a patient/client identifies with is part of which phase of MI?

   A. Engaging.
   B. Focusing.
   C. Evoking.
   D. Planning.

Correct Answer: A (Engaging).

Identifying gender pronouns in one of the first things an interviewer should inquire about to determine. Given that this task takes place during the initial phase of an interview, it is therefore part of the engagement phase of MI.

CHAPTER 10: TEACHING MOTIVATIONAL INTERVIEWING

1. Which of the following correctly pairs the name of the component of the Gradual Release of Responsibility Model with an accurate description?

   A. "I do it." SUPERVISION/FEEDBACK. Trainees are allowed time for independent practice and making mistakes. The trainer observes (in real time or after) use of the skills, solicits trainee input about the experience, reflects trainee feedback to the trainee, affirms skills well executed, and offers summaries. The trainer can also offer observations and opportunities for improvement as appropriate.

B. "We do it." COLLABORATION/MONITORING. The teacher participates with trainees in practicing skills, trainees practice the skill in a small group with the trainer leading the exercise, and trainees role-play among themselves, with the trainer listening and offering information and advice as appropriate.

C. "You do it." MODELING. The teacher introduces the skill, role-models the skill, provides examples, and demonstrates use.

D. "We do it." MODELING. The teacher introduces the skill, role-models the skill, provides examples, and demonstrates use.

Correct Answer: B ("We do it." COLLABORATION/MONITORING).

The other answer choices are incorrectly paired. "I do it" is paired with MODELING, "You do it" is paired with SUPERVISION/FEEDBACK.

2. Which of the following correctly pair a concept from the spirit of MI with an example of how to use it during MI training?

A. *Compassion*—Approaching the learners with an attitude that MI is easy to learn if you just memorize a few mnemonic devices and that practicing it once or twice is enough to be competent.

B. *Acceptance*—Understanding that your students have had training in how to talk to patients before and so they already know that MI can be useful to them and can see the benefit of working to develop good MI behaviors.

C. *Partnership*—Reminding your learners that you are the expert and so copying what you do is the only way to learn MI.

D. *Evocation*—Soliciting from learners, using open questions, their knowledge of MI and how they might find it useful.

Correct Answer: D (*Evocation*—Soliciting from learners, using open questions, their knowledge of MI and how they might find it useful).

Answer A is a common misconception about MI. Answer B may be a fair understanding, but it is not an example of Acceptance. Answer C is the opposite of the MI spirit of partnership.

3. Which of the following activities is a possible interactive exercise to practice focusing?

    A. *Agenda mapping:* Have participants split into groups of two. Draw
circles on a board or large piece of paper, and ask one partner to fill in
some with topics for discussion as part of the training agenda (e.g.,
common challenges when talking to clients or how to give feedback
in an MI-consistent way). Leave some empty circles, and then ask the
other person to fill in these circles. Have a collaborative discussion
about these topics and their significance, without choosing any particular focus yet. Then, on the basis of this discussion, ask an open-
ended question about which topic to start with first.

    B. *Drumming for change:* Prepare a list of statements, including prepara-
tory and mobilizing change talk, sustain talk, and other types of statements. Read each statement aloud. Instruct trainees to remain silent
if they hear sustain talk, to tap gently on their lap when they hear preparatory change talk (desire, ability, reason, need), and to drum loudly
or clap their hands when they hear mobilizing change talk (commitment, activation, and taking steps). Discuss any statements that have
a mixed response from the audience.

    C. *Snatching change talk from the jaws of ambivalence:* Prepare a list of state-
ments that include change talk embedded within at least two pieces
of sustain talk. Instruct your participants to select and then reflect the
change talk, rather than do a double-sided reflection.

    D. *Dodgeball:* Divide trainees into two teams. One team verbally "throws
out" resistance statements or sustain talk that they have heard. The other
team "dodges" resistance by responding in an MI-consistent manner
(with open questions, affirmations, reflections, and summaries). Teams
then switch roles. Have the larger group discuss examples that worked
well.

Correct Answer: A (Agenda mapping).

The other exercises could be used to practice the process of Evoking and
focus on change talk.

4. Ending MI training is best done by

    A. Completing a "real-play" full MI session with feedback from an ob-
server and the opportunity to practice in both the patient and clinician roles.

    B. Recording an actual MI session and then having an observer rate
your use of and adherence to MI.

C. Continually training, practicing, and using MI to maintain your proficiency.

D. Recognizing when you've acquired good MI skills and continuing to use these skills similarly in all patient encounters.

Correct Answer: C (Continually training, practicing, and using MI to maintain your proficiency).

Answers A and B may be good ways to conclude a training session. However, much MI training is an ongoing process of practicing and learning that should be adapted to the individual needs and situation of the person with whom you are working.

5. One tool that can be used to help evaluate and objectively assess use of MI is the

A. Special Education Against Resistance in MI Network (SpEAR MINt).

B. Motivational Interviewing Treatment Integrity (MITI) scale.

C. Motivational Interviewing Group Help Training Yield scale (MIGHTY scale).

D. Motivational Interviewing National Training Team Education Assistance (MINT TEA).

Correct Answer: B (Motivational Interviewing Treatment Integrity [MITI] scale).

The other scales and names do not (to our knowledge) exist.

CHAPTER 11: MOTIVATIONAL INTERVIEWING IN ADMINISTRATION, MANAGEMENT, AND LEADERSHIP

1. A Greek family rethinks its cooking strategies. On one hand, the health benefits of a lower-fat diet are well understood and appreciated. On the other, *fasolakia ladera* are not really *ladera* unless they happily swim in a sea of olive oil. Ambivalence and tension reign in the family. What's the stage of change?

A. Precontemplation.

B. Contemplation.

C. Preparation.

D. Action.

Correct Answer: B (Contemplation).

The family members actively consider their options and analyze the proposed change in terms of trade-offs between life with and life without *ladera*; they are in the contemplation stage of change. Given that ambivalence has been well established, the family system is past the precontemplation stage but has not yet resolved to take the next step in preparation for having a healthier diet.

2. After weeks of back-and-forth, your boss says: "I am trying to think of ways I can approve your salary increase by 20% as you are asking. One option is to expect more work from you, but I worry that my chief financial officer will not be too happy with the decision." What MI process does this case exemplify?

    A. Engaging.
    B. Focusing.
    C. Evoking.
    D. Planning.

Correct Answer: B (Focusing).

One aim of the focusing process is to help both parties feel comfortable in tolerating the uncertainty associated with change. In this case, you have been working hard to convince your boss that you deserve a raise. The boss's conditional approval, contingent on her increased expectations for your job performance, is an example of change talk. Such statements are openings for change. Your boss is already hinting at her own sources of ambivalence when the expected resistance by the company finance executive is mentioned.

3. Three friends are stranded in an elevator without their cell phones. One of them keeps buzzing the alarm bell and screams for help while another looks for a way out. The third friend waits for the other two to figure it out. This is an example of the

    A. Hawthorne effect.
    B. Pygmalion effect.
    C. Self-determination theory.
    D. Rumor transmission theory.

Correct Answer: C (Self-determination theory).

The self-determination theory of human motivation focuses on choices people make with their own free will: individual behavior is self-endorsed and self-determined. According to this theory, the three friends behave differently because of their autonomy. In contrast, social psychology theories, which form the basis for the Hawthorne and Pygmalion effects, point to environmental and social pressures as the main determinants of human behavior. According to social psychology, had we examined our subjects in a variety of social settings, we would be more impressed by the similarities than by the differences in the behavior of individuals under similar stressful conditions—such as being stranded in an elevator.

4. According to Jim Collins's analysis of successful companies, a leader's charisma is

    A. More likely to be a liability than an asset.
    B. More likely to be an asset than a liability.
    C. Irrelevant to success or failure.
    D. More important than the facts in motivating people.

Correct Answer: A (More likely to be a liability than an asset).

Charismatic leadership tends to promote a culture where the truth is not heard and the brutal facts are not confronted. An effective leader often succeeds despite his or her charisma—not because of it. Trying to motivate people on vision alone and ignoring the facts of the situation is a waste of time.

5. After having spent several months trying to convince your graphic designer to take 3-D courses in order to improve the quality of your products, he finally agrees. Two days later, he comes back and tells you that he changed his mind. Which of the following strategies will be most helpful in motivating him?

    A. Affirming one's strengths.
    B. Continued troubleshooting and recapitulation of goals.
    C. Following a guiding style.
    D. Developing discrepancies and resolving ambivalence.

Correct Answer: D (Developing discrepancies and resolving ambivalence).

During the evoking phase of MI, individuals often feel conflicted between allowing themselves to indulge in their motivation to change and the desire to maintain old habits and sustain the status quo. Developing discrepancies and resolving ambivalence facilitates change by fostering one's own motivation. In this example, you may find it helpful to explore the reasons behind your graphic designer's earlier motivation as well as stressors that might have contributed to him changing his mind.

Index

Page numbers printed in **boldface** *type refer to table or figures.*